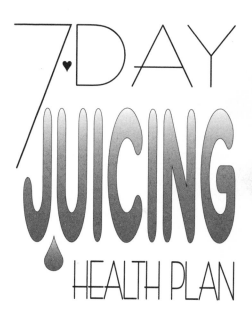

7 DAY JUICING HEALTH PLAN

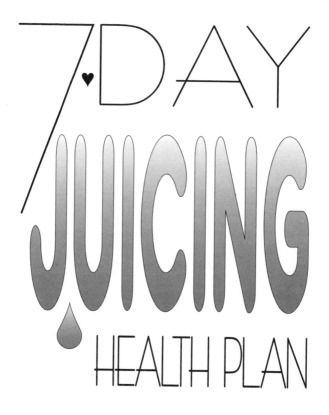

7 DAY JUICING HEALTH PLAN

Replace the missing elements in your diet

—— HELEN J. SIMPSON ——

foulsham

LONDON • NEW YORK • TORONTO • SYDNEY

foulsham

The Publishing House, Bennetts Close,
Cippenham, Slough, Berks SL1 5AP, England

*He bringeth forth grass for the cattle: and green
herb for the service of men.* Psalm 104:14

ISBN 0-572-02615-3

Printed in Great Britain by St. Edmundsbury Press, Bury St. Edmunds, Suffolk

CONTENTS

ACKNOWLEDGEMENTS

I wish to acknowledge the help given to me by the following people: Ann Bagnall of Southover Press, who continues to give me much encouragement and support; our nephew, soft fruit and apple grower Robert Simpson, for his advice and help; American food writer Bernard Clayton Jr, for permission to reproduce his recipe for Curried Pumpkin Soup; pharmacist Robert N. Gardiner, Dr Malcolm Lias. The Royal Society of Chemistry, for permission to use the vitamin and mineral data from their *Composition of Foods*. Dr Tom Sanders and Peter Bazalgette, co-authors of The Food Revolution; John Davidson of the Wholistic Research Company, for his information on buying juicers and for data from his *A Harmony of Science and Nature*; Brian Clements of the Hippocrates Health Centre, Florida, USA; nutrition scientist Dr Sarah Schenker of the British Nutrition Foundation; nutritionist Jackie Norton; Dr Robert Nash, research director of Molecular Nature Ltd; Annie Austin, Elizabeth Alderson and Amanda Howard. A very special thank you to Wendy Hobson, editorial director for my publishers W. Foulsham & Co. Ltd.

FOREWORD

We have known instinctively for centuries that a diet containing raw fruits and vegetables is essential to the body's health and well-being. Today, however, we tend to eat a high proportion of cooked and processed foods, and we know that because of the changing patterns of our lifestyle this is not always the healthiest diet. Drinking fresh juices made from raw fruits and vegetables as part of a sensible, balanced, wholefood diet is a brilliant way to change those old habits and set us on the path to a healthier and happier lifestyle.

We need to look again at the balance of our diet and how to give our bodies the best possible energy sources. We can learn a great deal from our ancestors about how a raw-energy diet can not only improve our health but also cure long-standing illnesses and prevent others from developing.

The diet of early peoples was high in vegetable matter, which consisted of the wild forms of the fruits and nuts we know today, together with watercress, fungi, the juicy roots of certain plants, and the larger and softer leaf buds. Even early civilisations were aware of the value of certain plants in the diet: in 500 BC Pythagoras recorded a cure for a weak digestion, which involved giving the patient nothing but mashed raw fruit, a little honey and goats' milk; almost 2,000 years ago, the Greek physician Dioscorides commended strawberry juice 'for cleansing the blood and major bodily organs of impurities, and for having a soothing effect on the temperament'. The Romans were exceedingly health conscious: the historian Pliny recorded the cultivation of plants for medical, dietary and aesthetic uses and if we look at the recipes of Apicius, who wrote the world's first-ever cookery book, we find healthy salads and delicious dressings.

In medieval times, highly nutritious salads using all kinds of fresh vegetables and herbs were prepared, as can be found in John Russell's *The Boke of Nurture*, published about 1460. In the seventeenth century John Evelyn created a salad garden at Saye Court in Deptford, with a calendar chart so that a fresh green salad could be served every day. He was one of the founding fathers of the English garden and was responsible for improving our vegetable gardens by promoting the cultivation of new and improved food plants from abroad. By the nineteenth century, generations of pioneers from Germany, Sweden and Switzerland were recording the healing effects of a diet rich in raw vegetables and fruits.

Although today many health professionals are taught that a weak digestive system finds it difficult to cope with raw foods, Max Bircher-Benner, the Swiss physician and pioneer of nutritional science, found raw apples highly beneficial in the treatment of digestive disorders and infections. His famous clinic in Zurich, founded in 1897, still flourishes today and advocates raw juice therapy among its treatments for serious illnesses.

Many outstanding medical and naturopath practitioners have used juice therapy. The German raw-food pioneer, Dr Max Gerson, cured cancer patients using chiefly the freshly made raw juices of fruits and vegetables high in potassium and other minerals. He also treated the great philosopher Albert Schweitzer, a severe diabetic taking huge doses of insulin, with a strict protein-free diet and a regime of raw and juiced fruit and vegetables. Despite their high sugar content, apples were also included in this treatment. After only one month on this specialised diet, Schweitzer needed no insulin at all and remained active and healthy until his death in 1956 at the age of 92.

Raw foods have an extraordinary capacity to promote a high level of health and alleviate a great deal of suffering in chronic illnesses. Cooking our food destroys much of its vitamin content, creates grievous losses of minerals and entirely eradicates enzymes that are essential to the efficient functioning of the body.

The sadness is that today many people are more concerned with accumulating wealth than concentrating on a good diet. Unfortunately we are at the mercy of a highly commercialised system of food processing and subjected to diverse water treatments. We know that some of these processes, such as fluoridation in water, can be beneficial, but equally that some processes introduced to food products may well be detrimental to human health. As a consequence of this adulteration, we are not eating a wholefood diet and are discarding many of the most important food elements. Eating too much processed food is bound to result in deficiencies of essential elements; too often convenience, colour effect and seasoning have become the overriding considerations at the expense of real nourishment.

It is therefore appropriate that many people are becoming more concerned with planning their daily meals around new dietary goals. These focus on a well-balanced, wholefood diet with the right balance of essential components such as vitamins and minerals, together with plenty of fibre, and natural rather than refined sugars, and foods low in sodium.

Diets containing fruit and vegetable juices are part of this phenomenon and sales of cookery books on fruit and vegetable juices are proving to be best-sellers. A wave of new juice bars is sweeping across both the USA and the UK to fortify health-conscious city workers. According to the American cookery writer, Bernard Clayton, millions of consumers are turning to such diets and the sale of home juicers has taken off. These powerful yet affordable machines produce invigorating juices, packed with vital nutrients, at the flip of a switch. We are being urged to 'juice it up'.

A recipe I found in an American juicer's cookbook just about sums it up: for one serving of a Peter Rabbit Special, you take a carrot, a celery stick, 3 Chinese leaves (stem lettuce), 4 sprigs of parsley and juice it up, adding a pinch of salt to taste, if needed. This simple drink contains a whole range of essential nutrients: carrots are packed with vitamins A and C, celery has significant amounts of calcium and other minerals, parsley is also rich in vitamins A and C plus calcium, potassium and magnesium-rich chlorophyll – and all are excellent digestive aids.

We have now entered a new millennium and leave behind the twentieth-century society which, in the developed world, is malnourished despite its wealth because of the rapid development in agricultural technologies. To the vast array of chemical and pharmaceutical products hidden in our food chain, and manufacturing processes that strip food of its nutritive value, we can now add the threat of genetically engineered foods – a topic we simply do not know enough about to be sure of its safety. Our diet has changed hugely in recent years to become fundamentally unhealthy, and yet we wonder why we suffer from increased mortality rates from heart disease, cancer, diabetes and other diet-related diseases. We know that in a health context prevention is always better than cure, so it makes sense for those who remain well to change their diet to a more healthy one and even those who are unfortunately facing the onslaught of a serious disease – who may wish they had changed a lifetime of unhealthy eating habits or given up smoking earlier – to embrace a new dietary regime.

With prevention in mind, I hope that through this book you will learn of the many health-giving properties that can be found in fruits, vegetables, herbs, grasses, sea vegetables, grains and pulses. The wisdom and science of nature, in all its plant forms, is God's gift to us on this planet. If we are to survive it is imperative that our eating patterns change. Encouragingly, scientists from all over the world are researching and discovering naturally occurring chemicals in living foods that can help to fight cancer and other diseases. We have this valuable knowledge and can put it to good use to change our eating habits. With this is in mind, it has been a real pleasure to devise the recipes in this book, all of which contain fruit and vegetable juices from the home juicer.

Happy juicing and good health.

Helen J. Simpson

AN INTRODUCTION TO JUICING

*Foods should be our medicine, and our medicine
should be our foods.*

Hippocrates, 359 BC

At last people are beginning to realise that our everyday diet is not as healthy as it should be because much of the nutritional value of food is destroyed by cooking, processing and preserving. Once you have acquired your home juicer you will be well on the way to a healthier and happier lifestyle, and you will soon discover the different and intense flavours and aromas found in freshly juiced fruit and vegetables, which you cannot obtain in the bottled, canned or concentrated juices.

I hope that through reading this book you will learn about all the essential nutrients that can be found in plant substances, which possess a wide range of active properties, including disease-preventive and therapeutic actions. Juices are great health builders and have the chemicals needed for tissue repair. As you consume these juices you should not only feel healthier but also acquire more energy and resistance to disease.

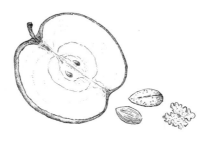

WHY JUICE?

The most obvious question to ask is why we should juice raw fruit and vegetables rather than eating them whole. The function of the home juicer is to extract the life-giving juice from the fibre even more efficiently than your own digestive system, and this cannot be compared with liquidisers or blenders, which merely purée foods. While fibre is obviously vital and must form a part of the overall diet, the major advantage of juicing is that the food is pulp-free and in this form the body can absorb the maximum quantity of essential nutrients directly into the bloodstream in minutes. Raw juices cannot be described as concentrated food, for a concentrated food is a product that has been dehydrated: they are liquid food in its natural state, composed of organic water of the highest quality, together with microscopic quantities of the atoms and molecules the body needs to stay alive.

Another question is why we need to juice fresh fruits and vegetables at home rather than buying juices. Fresh juices are bursting with living cells, free from additives and preservatives: canned, bottled and concentrated juices are pasteurised – or heated to achieve complete sterilisation – to increase their shelf life, which destroys many nutrients. In many cases, the manufactured products state that they contain 'added vitamin C' but in this case the vitamin serves only as an anti-oxidant and not as a nutrient (which we will explain in more detail later on). Another important point is that the ready-diluted fruit drinks that are often sold in cartons have no restriction on fruit or sugar content.

Soon after juicing the fruit or vegetable will deteriorate rapidly and begin to turn brown, which means it has oxidised and lost much of its nutritional value. For example, the act of slicing an orange causes it to lose some vitamin C, and apples begin to turn brown immediately after they have been cut. It is therefore important to consume juices immediately after juicing to obtain the maximum benefit. If you do have to store fresh juice, keep it in a thermos flask, preferably filled to the top so no air can get in, and store in the refrigerator for no more than 24 hours.

A HEALTHY BALANCED DIET

A diet comprising solely fruit and vegetable juice is **not** advocated. It is important to eat a balanced wholefood diet, and this should include daily fibre from fresh whole fruit and vegetables as well as pasta, rice, wholegrain cereals and home-made bread.

I recommend that you build up the juicing part of your diet slowly at first until you are consuming at least two 250 ml/8 fl oz/1 cup quantities of fresh fruit juice every day and, if possible, two similar-sized glasses of vegetable juice. The vegetable juices are the body builders and thus play a valuable part in your balanced diet.

The enzymes of fruits and vegetables are not compatible, so don't combine fruits and vegetables. The exception to this rule is apples, the only fruit that can be mixed with vegetable juices. Apples can also be used to clean out the juicer when switching between vegetable and fruit drinks.

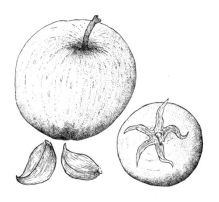

In *The Juiceman's Power of Juicing* (1992), Jay Kordich recommends that you chew vegetable juice and swirl it around in your mouth for 30–60 seconds before swallowing. He says: 'The warm juice stimulates and mixes with a digestive enzyme in the saliva called ptyalin (salivary amylase), which then accelerates digestion and absorption.' Kordich was heavily featured on American TV in the early 1990s and his flamboyant style conveyed to a large US audience a greater awareness of all the healthful properties that can be found in juiced fruits and vegetables, though some felt that his health claims were exaggerated. He had a lot to do with the increase in sales of home juicers and the juicing craze that swept the country. In other words, he put fun into juicing.

Juices are pure, natural and health-promoting and you can have great fun in your kitchen mixing them yourself. Of course, you can't squeeze a carrot for its juice by hand, so you will need a powerful machine to do the job! But I believe that in the twenty-first century a home juicer will become as essential a part of our everyday kitchen equipment as the microwave oven.

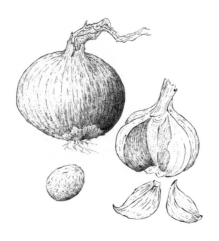

JUICERS AND JUICING EQUIPMENT

It is very important when buying a home juicer to consider the different types and sizes available. The power rating and capacity for juice yield will obviously dictate the price, and you tend to get what you pay for in efficiency. Ease of cleaning may be another consideration, and the level of noise and vibration in operation.

JUICE YIELDS

Many fruits and vegetables are around 85–95 per cent water, with nutrients in solution, the remaining percentage being the solids – fibrous and cell-wall materials. So, with efficiency in mind, you need to choose a juicer that extracts the most nutrients from the solids.

There are two types of home juicer available: the cheaper centrifugal juicers and the more powerful and efficient masticating models.[1] Many popular centrifugal juicers merely grate the fruit or vegetables, using a high-speed shredder, so the fibres and cell walls are not adequately broken up to produce a top-quality juice. A masticating juicer, on the other hand – such as the Champion or Green Power Super Plus Juice Extractor – chews the fibres and breaks up the cells of fruit and vegetables. This results in more fibre, enzymes, vitamins and trace minerals in the finished juice, which will have a darker, richer colour and a sweeter, richer, more full-bodied flavour. You will also have up to 25 per cent more juice containing three times as many cell nutrients extracted and, if you combine this with a juice press – such as the Health Stream Press – you can extract a further 300 per cent. The Green Power Super Plus Juice Extractor will also juice fibrous plants such as wheatgrass, culinary herbs, alfalfa and other sprouts, but it does not have as

---

[1] The source of much of this material is John and Lucie Davidson, *A Harmony of Science and Nature*, Wholistic Research Co, 1999.

wide a feed-in chamber as the Champion, so a large carrot would have to be quartered before juicing. The Champion has a faster speed of juicing and is easier to clean and assemble. However, both models will make nut butters, purées (pastes), baby foods, desserts and frozen fruit sorbets.

CENTRIFUGAL JUICERS

There are two types of centrifugal juicer: some are separators, which operate without needing to be cleaned out and therefore give you continuous processing; others are batch operators which have to be cleaned out every 900 g/2 lb of material being juiced, so you need to stop, empty the pulp container basket and start again.

If you decide on a batch operator, you may need to look for a larger-capacity model that will not need emptying after providing only two or so glasses of juice when you are serving several people.

Centrifugal juicers contain a steel or aluminium basket with mesh at the sides and blades at the bottom that rotate as fast as the machine's motor will allow. Look for the most robust model with the strongest motor.

Fruits and vegetables are shredded by the blades and the juice passes through the mesh while the pulp is spun out into a separate basket. Some machines have wider holes than others for inserting the fruits and vegetables; if the hole is too small, you may have to cut up larger vegetables before you can fit them in.

Choose a juicer that is easy to assemble and take apart as all juicers have to be washed after every use. Many centrifugal juicers use aluminium discs and baskets, which some believe to be a poisonous metal.

The following machines are all available in the UK and most retail from about £39 to £150. They are all BEAB approved and have passed electrical safety tests.

Makers of centrifugal juicers in America include Acme, Braun, Juiceman, Olympic, Oster, Panasonic, Phoenix, Salton and Sanyo.

KENWOOD
The Kenwood 500 and 600 models both have two speeds: one for soft fruits, the other for harder fruits and vegetables. The jug supplied with the 500 has a foam separator, but the more powerful 600 is more substantial in operation. The juice capacity is 500 ml/17 fl oz/2¼ cups (about three glasses). They are widely available and cost £40–45.

MOULINEX
The Moulinex 753 is their top-of-the-range model, which has a large 1.3 litre/2¼ pt/5¼ cup capacity, and this model gives you continuous processing. It is easy to clean and widely available at about £40.

BRAUN
The Braun Multipress Automatic MP80 (4290) is a batch operator and has a useful feed-in tray that can double as a dust cover. Its capacity is 450 ml/¾ pt/2 cups (about three glasses). The manufacturers advise against juicing redcurrants and blackcurrants. It is easy to clean and widely available at about £40.

PHILIPS
The Philips Licuardora HR 2820, like the Braun, has a useful feed-in tray. The capacity is 600 ml/1 pt/2½ cups (three to four glasses). It is available in major stores for around £50. The Phillips Juice 7 Co. HR1840 is a one power-unit centrifugal juicer that incorporates a blender. It is easy to clean but its white plastic is prone to discolouring. About £45 from Selfridges, London (0207 629 1234).

MAGIMIX
The Magimix Le Duo Divertimento is a combined juice extractor and citrus press and has a heavy-duty metal basket. It is quiet and easy to clean. £99.95 (£20 extra for chrome) mail order (0181 246 4300).

VITAMINE
The stainless steel Vitamine Rotal Automatic Fruit and Vegetable Juicer is quick, easy and continuous. £148 from the Wholistic Research Co. (01707 262686; fax 01707 258828).

WARING
The PJE50 model is a top-of-the-range stainless steel juice extractor. £239 from Harrods, John Lewis and Conran shops.

MASTICATING JUICERS

As we have said, masticating juicers, though more expensive than centrifugal juicers, extract a greater quantity of juice and less pulp from the produce, resulting in a much more nutritious drink. Some models have a double-screw mechanism that crushes the produce to a paste rather than shredding it, then squeezes the juice through a screen in the bottom. In the case of the Champion model a single cutter with many teeth rotates inside a stainless steel-lined body, breaking up all the cells. The Green Power Super Plus model has a twin-gear crushing system.

THE CHAMPION
A highly recommended powerful and robust machine, suitable for commercial use. It comes with an attachment for nut butters and sorbets etc. but the grain and coffee mill attachment is extra. 5-year guarantee. £299 from the Wholistic Research Co. (01707 262686; fax 01707 258828).

GREEN POWER
The Super Plus Juice Extractor deserves serious consideration. It's perfect for fibrous plants such as wheatgrass – it even juices pine needles! It makes nut butters, purées (pastes), baby foods, desserts and frozen fruit sorbets. It has a pasta attachment. A specialist juicer but slower than the Champion (some users might be happier with a Champion model and a manual wheatgrass juicer). £399 from the Wholistic Research Co. (01707 262686; fax 01707 258828).

GREEN LIFE

The Green Life Juice Extractor is a similar machine to the Champion but can also juice wheatgrass to make a powerful chlorophyll-rich juice, as well as juicing fruits and vegetables. £390 from Savant distribution (0113 230 1993).

WHEATGRASS OR SLOW-TURNING JUICERS

These slow-turning juicers operate in a completely different way from high-speed juicers. The motor slowly turns a blade inside the juicer, which presses the juices from leafy green vegetables, sprouting plants, wheatgrass and soft vegetables, rather than masticating them in the high-speed machines. If you plan to make all the recipes for juices listed in this book, especially wheatgrass and alfalfa juice, you will need both a high-speed and a low-speed juicer.

GREEN LEAF

A manual juicer that works like an old-fashioned hand mincer. It is elegantly designed in stainless steel and is easy to use and clean. £159 from the Wholistic Research Co. (01707 262686; fax 01707 258828).

HEALTH FOUNTAIN

Another manual juicer, and a standard item in many American natural health centres. It is specially for juice extraction from wheatgrass and other fibrous or difficult-to-juice plant materials, including bean and other sprouts. £89 from the Wholistic Research Co. (01707 262686; fax 01707 258828).

PORKET

The Porket manual juicer is a cheap alternative to the Health Fountain and Green Leaf manual juicers, and is made in the Czech Republic. It is tin-plated and therefore care is needed to avoid rusting, otherwise it performs well. £34.95 from the Wholistic Research Co. (01707 262686; fax 01707 258828).

JUICE PRESSES

After using a centrifugal or masticating juicer, the resulting pulp will still be moist but by then using a manual or motorised juice press the pulp can be further processed to yield over 90 per cent of available juice. You are left with a flat pancake of reduced solids resembling a piece of cardboard!

HEALTH STREAM

The Health Stream Manual Juice Press comes with a stainless steel juicing pan and beechwood pressing block. It can be used with most regular juicers to provide 25–200 per cent more juice with a very high nutritional content. The new 4-tonne model is £278. The Health Stream Motorised Hydraulic Juice Press is as above but motorised with automated press-button operation. £1,995. Both models are available from the Wholistic Research Co. (01707 262686; fax 01707 258828).

CITRUS JUICERS

The following manufacturers also make juicers specifically for citrus fruits: Braun, Kenwood, Krups, Moulinex and Philips.

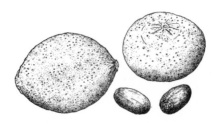

STORING AND CLEANING YOUR HOME JUICER

It is a good idea to keep your juicer in a prominent place near the kitchen sink, with a large space for cutting vegetables and fruit on a board nearby. The machine should be stored with the cable safely away from the sink and it and your knives should be kept away from young children.

If you are to become a serious home-juicer, you'll also need to store large quantities of fresh fruits and vegetables, perhaps attractively displayed in big, colourful bowls.

You'll be using your juicer every day so make sure you empty the pulp as soon as possible from the large receptacle or odours may develop and tiny fruit flies may appear, especially in hot weather. The pulp can be used in many baking recipes (see pages 170–6) and also makes excellent garden compost. It is not necessary to clean the juicer between juicing different types of juice; simply juice an apple to clear the way for new juices, whether fruit or vegetable. However, you should clean it after every juicing session, otherwise the pulp will harden and make cleaning more difficult.

Switch off and unplug the juicer before dismantling the parts for cleaning. The removable parts can be rinsed under running water – a spray or hairwashing hose attached to the sink taps will help. You don't need detergents as there are no oils or sticky sugars to remove. The stainless steel centrifugal filter basket usually requires a little scrubbing with a brush or soft pad.

Every few days soak the removable parts in a solution of two parts dishwasher detergent to one part bleach in a sink full of hot water. Leave them overnight and you will find carrot and other stains will disappear without rubbing. Thoroughly rinse the parts in clean water before drying and reassembling the juicer ready to use again.

OTHER JUICING EQUIPMENT

- Polyethylene cutting boards: many people use colour-coded boards – green for fruit, brown for vegetables
- Kitchen scales
- A sturdy bristled scrubbing brush to clean vegetables and fruit before juicing
- High-quality chopping knives, which need to be sharpened regularly
- A peeler for paring some produce ready for juicing when the pulp is also needed (some vegetables such as carrots should not be peeled as there's so much goodness in the skins)
- A calibrated measuring jug
- A salad spinner for removing excess water from washed vegetables
- A strainer for straining juices if required
- A large lidded storage jug suitable for use in the refrigerator
- Glass storage bowls with plastic lids
- Zipped plastic bags for storing washed and dried vegetables
- A blender for mixing juices with fruit purées, yoghurt, milk, water, honey or added wheatgerm etc., and for blending bananas, avocados, apricots etc. with prepared juices and mixing salad dressings, soups and sauces

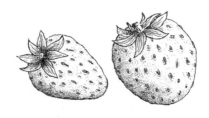

DOS AND DON'TS OF JUICING

Before embarking on juicing, it is important to note a few of the following dos and don'ts for safety and to ensure long service from your juicer.

PRODUCTS

- Support your local economy and environment by finding a local fruit and vegetable farm, though I do not believe that organic foods are necessarily safer or more nutritious than inorganic.[2]
- Buy produce in bulk where appropriate. For example, you could buy freshly dug carrots by the sackload, which you can then wash and store until needed in a cool dark place. (A second refrigerator in a garage would also be very useful for storage.)
- Buy unwaxed English apples so the whole apple can be put through the juicer.

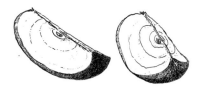

---

[2] Some American books on juicing have reported that non-organic produce is potentially harmless. On the subject of Alar (a chemical – no longer used in Britain – to increase the yield on trees and stop apples falling too early) and other chemicals, Peter Bazalgette states: 'There is no evidence for this whatsoever. Washing apples is a good idea because some are just plain dirty. But there is no danger from pesticide or even fungicide washes (that are most commonly found in citrus fruit). To put it simply – there is more danger from the cyanide in the pips than from chemicals ... and there is no danger from the pips!'

- Wash all fruits and vegetables thoroughly as soon as possible after purchase. Use a vegetable scrubbing brush if necessary.
- Don't peel carrots before juicing: washing them well instead means you will receive the maximum nutrition from the whole vegetable.
- Most fruits and vegetables can be juiced along with their peel, seeds and stems to obtain optimum nutrition.[3] Oranges and grapefruits, however, should be peeled but juiced with as much of the white pith as possible. (Whole lemons and limes can be juiced entirely.)
- Use a salad spinner to remove excess water from green vegetables.
- Store washed and dried prepared produce in a refrigerator or in a cool dark place in sealed plastic bags ready for use.
- When preparing vegetables and fruit for juicing, slice or dice them immediately before they are to be juiced and drunk, for vitamin C losses are high on exposure to air.

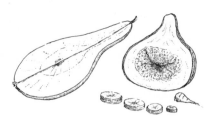

---

[3] In a letter to me, Peter Bazalgette states: 'There is no danger from pips pressed into apple juice. There is only a minute amount of cyanide, and it is soon dissipated into the juice. Only if someone made quantities of paste exclusively from pips could a problem arise.' (Some people, however, prefer to discard apple pips before juicing as they tend to turn the juice slightly brown.)

JUICING TECHNIQUES

- Don't force the produce through the juicer: feed it in slowly.
- Either cut up carrots into 5–7.5 cm/2–3 in pieces or feed the large end in first.
- Bunch up greens together in clumps and put them through with a pusher.
- Pears can be used if firm and ripe. Juice the pieces alternately with apple pieces, starting and ending with a piece of apple.
- Do not try to juice bananas, apricots or figs. Use a blender instead and thin down with other juices or milk.
- Insert juicy fruits such as melons and watermelons slowly, in order to obtain a larger quantity of juice.

SAFETY

- The safety interlock mechanism found on the side catches of most models ensures that the machine can be operated only when the lid is firmly in position.
- Do not allow children to operate or play with the juicer.
- Never use your fingers to push food into the hopper, and food should always be fed in with the motor in operation.

CONSUMING JUICES

- Fruits and vegetables should not be combined – their enzymes are not compatible – except for apples, which can be mixed with vegetable juices and can also be used to clean out the juicer when switching between vegetable and fruit drinks.
- Don't drink green juices (i.e. spinach, parsley, lettuce, Brussels sprouts, cabbage and kale) or beetroot (red beet) juices alone. Such a mixture could be too potent and cause gastric discomfort. These juices should always be diluted in a ratio of one part green or beetroot juice to three parts apple or carrot juice or mineral water. (This does not apply to celery or cucumber juices.)

- Don't mix melon juices with other fruits. They contain different enzymes, which are difficult to digest when mixed.
- It is advisable to drink fresh juices on an empty stomach, either half an hour before a meal or half an hour after, or as a between-meal snack to avoid digestive upsets. This is because the juices can ferment while the digestive tract deals with other food in the stomach.
- It is also advisable to wait between drinking different juices: after drinking a fruit juice, wait at least one minute before consuming a vegetable juice; and allow at least 10 minutes after drinking a vegetable juice before consuming a fruit juice.
- You should always dilute vegetable and fruit juices for children with water as the neat juices are too potent for young digestive systems. Teenagers should restrict themselves to one or two 150 ml/¼ pt/⅔ cup glasses of raw juices a day.
- If you are diabetic or have any other medical condition, consult your doctor before embarking on a fruit-juice programme. Although small quantities of unsweetened fruit juices can be included in a diabetic diet, it must be counted as part of the carbohydrate allowance. Too much fresh fruit juice instead of fruit should not be relied on as it doesn't contain any of the important fibre that is present in the whole fruit for diabetics. It may, therefore, be wise to keep to vegetable juices.

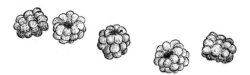

7-DAY JUICING HEALTH PLAN

It is important to begin slowly with a juicing diet and to combine it with a sensible everyday diet. The juicing programme can be increased when your stomach and digestive system have adjusted to the new regime.

Eating patterns have changed and three meals a day is now a thing of the past; except when entertaining, meals today are largely quick and easy. Much depends on your budget and how much time you want to spend in the kitchen. Colour, texture and flavour all help to make food and drink enjoyable, and there is an enormous range of all three in juiced fruit and vegetable drinks.

For many working people the main meal of the day is eaten in the evening, but the following day-by-day menu plan gives lunch time as the main meal to allow plenty of time for digestion (a large cooked evening meal can often lead to disturbed sleep). Meals should fit in with our lifestyles: there are no hard and fast rules for individuals as to when to eat or even how much to eat, but eating at regular intervals of 5–6 hours, with no in-between snacks, is recommended. However, this does exclude diabetics, who may require snacks at certain times of the day to boost their blood sugar levels, and children and the elderly, who may not be able to consume large quantities at one meal and need snacks to boost their calorie and nutrient intake. In these cases, the vegetable drinks taken mid- or late afternoon will be an excellent pick-me-up.

Rather than relying on workplace canteens or food from shops, cafés, sandwich bars and pubs, which are often high in fat and low in fibre, working people can take in their own lunches – an effective way in controlling what you eat at midday. If you have a refrigerator or microwave at work, you can increase the range of options from prepared sandwiches to include salads and home-made soups and juiced drinks in a thermos flask. A home freezer provides an excellent opportunity to cook extra quantities of foods as standbys for busy working people.

At long last nutritionists have changed the traditional food wheel, which outlined four food groups (meat, dairy, vegetables/fruit and grains) that formed a building block for our daily eating habits. The new food wheel below suggests a diet high in grains, fruits and vegetables, with lower amounts of milk, yoghurt, cheese, meats, nuts, fats and sweets. According to Brian Clement, director of the Hippocrates Health Institute in West Palm Springs, Florida, the reason why so many Americans are still hooked on meat and dairy products is because 'Today's nutritional attitudes are dictated by commercial industries that support only what is profitable. Meat and dairy products make big money; vegetables, fruits, grains, seeds and nuts do not.'[4] My main argument with his 'living foods' diet, however, is its lack of warmth nourishment, which is so essential in the northern European climate.

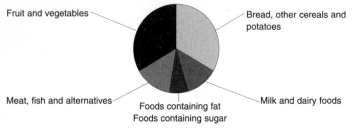

Fruit and vegetables

Bread, other cereals and potatoes

Meat, fish and alternatives

Foods containing fat
Foods containing sugar

Milk and dairy foods

My menu plan is not vegetarian based, but is designed as a 'go-between' diet. There are hundreds of ways to be a vegetarian. For example, the vegan diet, with its strictly prohibited foods (meat, fish, poultry, eggs and dairy products), must make sure that there are no vitamins and mineral lacking and that it provides enough calories. There are benefits and risks to be considered in both vegetarian and omnivore diets, and neither can claim to have a monopoly on healthy eating. Similar health benefits can be gained from both well-selected omnivorous and vegetarian diets.

The fruit and vegetable variety of cocktails in my diet should be consumed at least half an hour before eating, or they can be replaced by simply juicing two or three oranges before breakfast, or three carrots for the mid-afternoon booster. Both will supply you with plenty of vitamins and minerals.

---

[4] From Clement and Digeronimo's enlightened and readable *Living Foods for Optimum Health,* Prima, 1998.

This plan is based on about 2,000 calories per day, with a daily allowance of 300 ml/½ pt/1¼ cups of skimmed milk per day, to be used in breakfast cereals, tea or coffee. I have also allowed for a traditional English-style breakfast on day 6. Of course, you can switch around the meals if you wish as long as you maintain a healthy balance.

DAY ONE

Fruit juice	No 14: Morning Pick-up (see page 126)
Breakfast	Grilled mushrooms and poached egg 2 slices of wholemeal toast with polyunsaturated margarine and marmalade
Lunch	Roast chicken, jacket potato, boiled carrots, broccoli or beans and skimmed gravy Baked apple and custard
Vegetable juice	No 14: Carrot and Apple Juice Lifesaver (see page 148)
Dinner	Watercress soup Mashed sardine and cottage cheese bap Banana

DAY TWO

Fruit juice	No 4: Apple and Orange Juice (see page 121)
Breakfast	A bowl of bran flakes with 150 ml/¼ pt/⅔ cup semi-skimmed milk from allowance A slice of wholemeal toast with mashed banana
Lunch	Baked trout served with a thin lemon sauce, new potatoes, and French (green) beans or peas Plums cooked in orange juice and served with natural yoghurt
Vegetable juice	No 2: Winter's Tonic (see page 142)
Dinner	Vegetarian lasagne with a cauliflower, watercress, (bell) pepper and walnut or mushroom and chive salad Wholemeal roll

DAY THREE

Fruit juice	No 6: Hawaiian Sunrise (see page 122)
Breakfast	Boiled egg 2 slices of wholemeal toast with polyunsaturated margarine and marmalade
Lunch	Lancashire hot-pot with peas, cabbage or mashed swede (rutabaga) Fresh fruit salad
Vegetable juice	No 4: Broccoli Surprise (see page 143)
Dinner	Vegetable soup Jacket potato filled with grated cheese Orange and Date Wholemeal Loaf (see page 176) A slice of cantaloupe melon

DAY FOUR

Fruit juice	No 9: Strawberry Fayre (see page 124)
Breakfast	A bowl of unsweetened muesli and 150 ml/¼ pt/⅔ cup semi-skimmed milk from allowance A slice of wholemeal bread and a slice of lean ham
Lunch	Salmon risotto made with brown rice, sliced green (bell) pepper and onion Green salad Apple and Date Compôte (see page 169) with 200 ml/7 fl oz/scant 1 cup Greek-style yoghurt
Vegetable juice	No 6: Peter Rabbit's Delight (see page 144)
Dinner	Chicken soup Mashed sardine and cottage cheese granary bap Nectarine or peach

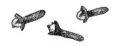

DAY FIVE

Fruit juice	No 7: Kiwi Medley (see page 123)
Breakfast	Porridge with chopped banana and 150 ml/¼ pt/⅔ cup semi-skimmed milk from allowance A slice of wholemeal toast with marmalade or low-sugar lemon curd
Lunch	Fish pie with peas, beans and courgettes (zucchini) A slice of melon
Vegetable juice	No 8: Apple Aniseed (see page 145)
Dinner	Leek and potato soup Pitta bread filled with tuna, prawns (shrimp), cottage cheese and shredded lettuce Raspberry sorbet

DAY SIX

Fruit juice	No 21: Tropical Cancer Fighter (see page 130)
Breakfast	2 rashers (slices) grilled (broiled) lean back bacon, 2 grilled tomato halves, 1 poached egg 2 slices of wholemeal toast with polyunsaturated margarine and marmalade
Lunch	2 small grilled lamb or pork chops, trimmed of all fat with Apple Mustard Sauce (see page 167), jacket potato, peas, French (green) beans and skimmed gravy A slice of melon
Vegetable juice	No 9: The Body Builder (see page 146)
Dinner	75 g/3 oz (dried weight) tagliatelle, boiled and served with a caper and walnut sauce Summer pudding or melon and strawberry salad

Fruit juice	No 5: Minted Apple and Blood Orange Juice (see page 121)
Breakfast	2 shredded wheat or weetabix with chopped apple, raisins and walnuts and semi-skimmed milk from allowance A slice of wholemeal toast with a thin scraping of yeast extract
Lunch	Roast beef and a portion of Yorkshire pudding, or roast lamb with onion and mint sauce, with 2 roast potatoes or boiled new potatoes, and sprouts, broccoli, green beans or grated carrots seasoned and baked in 15 ml/1 tbsp water, 15 ml/1 tbsp lemon juice and a knob of butter in a slow oven Cheesecake made with yoghurt and low-fat cheese or fruit marinated in liqueurs with low-fat yoghurt
Vegetable juice	No 11: The Body Cleanser (see page 147)
Dinner	Minestrone soup Ham and watercress wholemeal sandwich Fresh fruit

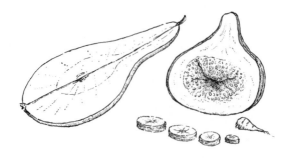

SLIMMING WITH THE HOME JUICER

It has been said that half the population of Britain is overweight, and half of those are obese. Ordinary slimming diets are notoriously poor nutritionally, and diets of cooked foods, vitamin pills and food supplements will never be as beneficial to your system as raw juice dieting.

Some cancer research studies have shown that people who are 40 per cent or more above their ideal weight appear to have a higher cancer risk. However, it is not known whether it is the extra pounds or the types of food eaten that are responsible for this risk. A 12-year study in the United States indicated that marked obesity was linked to higher death rates from cancers of the gall bladder, kidney, stomach, colon, breast and the lining of the uterus when compared with people of normal weight. The World Cancer Research Fund encourages eating low-calorie, nutrient-rich foods such as fruits, vegetables, grain cereals and pulses as alternatives to calorie-laden, high-fat foods. The juices of fruits and vegetables can be a very important part of such a programme.

A planned juicing diet to achieve a desirable body weight can be organised alongside a balanced calorie intake and physical activity. Successful slimming is not achieved overnight but is a long-term process. To be effective, weight loss should be slow and gradual. Dieters who stop and start diets all the time often end up with their bodies containing a higher proportion of body fat than when they first started dieting. This has been called the 'yo-yo effect', and may be more harmful to health than being slightly overweight. Weight loss should mean losing fat and not other body stores, such as protein from the muscles, but as fat is the body's long-term storage it is the hardest energy store to reduce.

HOW MANY CALORIES?

The Department of Health and Social Security recommends that an average woman requires approximately 2,200 calories a day, and a man requires approximately 3,000 calories a day to maintain weight. However some recent research suggests that these levels may be too high, and some normal-weight women require only 1,850 calories, with the same decreased proportion for men. Studies of overweight people show that the majority of women lose weight on a 1,000–1,200 calorie diet and most men lose weight on 1,200–1,500 calories a day. An excellent target is a loss of 0.9–1.75 kg/2–4 lb a week for the first two or three weeks and 0.45–0.9 kg/1–2 lb per week thereafter. This is the equivalent of 500–1,000 calories less than would normally be eaten a day.

EXERCISE

It is now recognised that exercise is almost as important as the diet itself. Exercise certainly speeds the process and tones up the muscles, which ultimately improves body shape and increases the suppleness, stamina and strength of the body. People forget that the heart is a muscle and like most muscles needs exercise.

Exercise need not be over-strenuous initially. Regular aerobic classes, swimming, running, jogging, dancing, trampolining, cycling and digging the garden are all good forms of exercise.

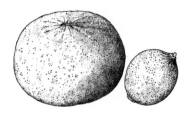

FAD DIETS

Remember that the slimming business is a very profitable one. Unfortunately, only a minority of diets are sensible and even these often do not succeed; some diets are nutritionally inadequate as they do not provide enough vitamins and minerals; and some diets even constitute a health risk. Fasting and very severe dieting can cause nausea, vomiting, fatigue, dizziness and low blood pressure and even lead to severe depression and irritability. Unbalanced diets have been criticised by orthodox doctors and dieticians: for example, a highly dangerous liquid protein diet combined with fasting in the 1970s in the USA was believed to have caused at least sixty deaths.

Dieting can be easy to start but sometimes difficult to keep up, and success is possible only if your new way of eating becomes part of a permanent change in lifestyle. Set yourself realistic goals: if you need to shed two stones, concentrate on the first stone before tackling the next. Learn to say a polite no to food outside your diet plan that is offered to you. Try to be hungry at meal times, and if you aren't hungry at meal times eat a bit less, or perhaps have a little extra at the next meal. There will be times when you want to cheat, but try to keep occupied: some slimmers brush their teeth every time they want to eat, others play patience or take up knitting!

Only weigh yourself once or twice a week because your weight fluctuates through the day due to changes in water retention and disappointing readings can be discouraging. After you have been dieting for a while your weight may seem to remain stationery; this happens as your body gets used to receiving less food and adjusts to a slower metabolism.

THE JUICING DIET

As with any weight reduction diet, it is advisable to check with your doctor before beginning a regime that includes a lot of juices.

Raw juice slimming does not mean starvation and it is a great way to lose weight naturally without feeling deprived of food. It means super nutrition and, with regular exercise, it is a safe, slow, steady way to reach permanent weight loss. It has been said that the same raw food diet prescribed in the health clinics of Europe to treat cancer, diabetes and arthritis can work wonders for the overweight. Health farms continue to heal and rejuvenate their clients with fresh raw juices, but at a price: a home juicer in your kitchen can provide the same benefits and at far less expense.

'Living' food juices vibrate – giving you a sense of well-being – and fresh raw juices provide you with instant raw energy, a tonic 'pick me up'. The late Dr Norman Walker also said that dieting on juices gives you the highest density of nutrients for calorie intake and the lowest fat intake of any diet, and it is the easiest, most comfortable way to lose a few pounds. When overtaxed by stress and obesity, raw juices restore normal responsiveness to the adrenal glands, improve your muscle tone and, most importantly, process the entire body through a spring cleaning, giving your digestive machine a chance to rest.

Simply substitute a glass of juice for one of your daily meals, say lunch, and eat your regular breakfast and dinner menu. This way you should lose 3.5–4.5 kg/8–10 lb a month. Weight gain can happen over several years and it is, therefore, very wise to slim slowly with a sensible diet. Consuming fruit and vegetable juices softens the pangs of hunger and once embarked on a juice programme for slimming your desire for fattening and sweet foods will disappear. You can always dilute pure fruit juice with a little water to reduce its acidity.

Carrot, spinach, beetroot (red beet) and cucumber juices are especially recommended for a slimming programme. Make a quantity of carrot juice, approximately 175 ml/6 fl oz/¾ cup, and combine it with 60–90 ml/2–3 fl oz of any of the other three. See pages 141–152 for more ideas for delicious and appetising vegetable juice combinations.

A 250 ml/8 fl oz/1 cup glass of fruit juice contains about l00 calories, a glass of vegetable juice about half that amount. Drinking a glass of juice mid-morning and another mid-afternoon will also help quell any hunger pains. It is advisable when weight watching not to exceed more than six glasses of juice a day, because large quantities of unsweetened fruit juices shouldn't be drunk on a diet. The calorie content of a small glass (100 ml/ 3½ fl oz/scant 1 cup) of fruit juice is approximately 50 kilocalories, therefore 1 litre/1¾ pts/4¼ cups of fresh fruit juice would contain approximately 500 kilocalories – which is half a day's calorie allowance for slimmers.

Why not wean your partner from some of those calorie-packed business lunches and offer instead a flask of a freshly juiced fruit or vegetable drink, with perhaps a wholemeal sandwich. The evening meal will be appreciated far more and he or she will be happier and healthier for having shed a few pounds. Simply place an ice cube in the thermos, freshly juice a drink and fill the flask to the very top, ready for a snack or picnic!

It is worth mentioning that one of the most successful and disease-reducing diets in the world today is the Mediterranean diet. It consists of olive oil (used sparingly), pasta, cereals, potatoes and rice, freshly dressed salads, fish and lean meat, large quantities of fresh fruit and vegetables, and garlic, which is now said to inhibit cancer growth. Freshly juiced fruits and vegetables can be very much a part of this healthy Mediterranean diet.

THE BENEFITS OF RAW JUICE FASTING

Raw juice fasting is one of the best ways to eliminate harmful toxins and accumulated wastes that can build up because of stress or poor nutrition. It is now common practice in addiction centres to steer people off alcohol and drugs by placing them on a detoxification programme.

The cleansing period of raw juice fasting can be recommended over a one-, two- or three-day period. A longer period of fasting is not advocated because you are likely to succumb to the need to catch up on lost food supply and consequently you can soon return to your original weight or maybe increase it. Those suffering from serious conditions such as diabetes or blood diseases should never attempt fasting. Elderly people should always seek medical advice before following a fasting programme. Fasting on water alone can also be dangerous, but it is important to make sure you drink at least 2.25–3.5 litres/4–6 pts/10–15 cups of liquid each day because of the dangers of dehydration.

When raw juice fasting, substitute for each meal one or two 250 ml/8 fl oz/1 cup quantities of vegetable or fruit juice, which can be diluted with mineral water. Remember to drink your vegetable drink first, and wait ten minutes before consuming a fruit juice. You can also make up the liquid quantity during the day with lemon and water sweetened with a little honey.

The main purpose of juice fasting is to restore the body to a healthy state. The Swiss *rohsaft kur* (raw juice cure) is used worldwide by leading health spas, with the knowledge that it can reduce high blood pressure, and high cholesterol and uric acid levels in your bloodstream. Pounds can be shed in the process, and the skin clears and tightens. Nails become healthier and stronger, hair develops a shine and the eyes brighten. The digestive organs benefit from the rest, and the patient feels more mentally alert and active.

On the subject of a detoxing programme, it should be noted that almost a third of the body's waste products are eliminated through the skin. The health specialist Leslie Kenton recommends spending five minutes a day dry-brushing our bodies with a long-handled natural bristle brush or a rough hemp glove as an important measure to rid our bodies of harmful toxins and encourage better lymphatic circulation. With the exception of your face, brush the entire body with the dry brush or glove. For maximum benefit, take a warm shower afterwards, then switch to a 30-second cold only shower. Dry yourself and keep warm. This is an excellent method for cellulite-prone women to rid themselves of harmful toxins, though a radical change in diet and lots of exercise is also needed.

It is important to keep your fast days free and only do things that require a limited amount of energy and effort. Read a good book. If you feel the need to sleep then do so. In general, try to relax and if possible include plenty of fresh air during the day.

When breaking the fast, return to solid food gradually and then, when your body and stomach has adjusted to this new regime, return to your normal diet.

We spend a fortune on grooming and cleansing and looking after our external bodies and spare very little thought about the cleansing of the colon. Good colon health is vital to our everyday well-being. Although some people manage to go without passing a stool for several days, it is best for your body to have a bowel movement at least once a day, so that toxins are not collecting for too long. It is said that it takes 8–12 hours for food to be fully digested, and for all the nutrients to be absorbed, and for the waste to be eliminated. The late Dr Norman Walker stated that colon neglect is the cause of many deaths. He described the colon as 'the body's sewer' and constipation as 'our bodies' greatest enemy'.[5]

Many health centres and health care providers practice giving full enemas, as being the quickest and easiest way to unblock a congested colon of the sticky debris sent from all parts of the body for elimination. However, I have my reservations about the use of enemas and even more about the very drastic methods of colonic irrigations used by chiropractors, physical therapists and even physicians. Colonic irrigation is expensive, the process can be very

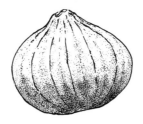

---

[5] Norman W. Walker, *Colon Health: the Key to Vibrant Life.*

uncomfortable, and sometimes the presence of the tube can induce severe cramps and pain. There have been cases where the equipment has not been adequately sterilised between treatments and where germs have passed from one patient to another, and at least six patients in America died following bowel perforation. It appears that no license or training is required to operate colonic irrigation devices.[6]

Constipation can usually be remedied more naturally by increased fibre content in the diet, and increased water intake and regular exercise. Only a doctor should be consulted if constipation persists or if a patient recognises a significant change in bowel patterns.

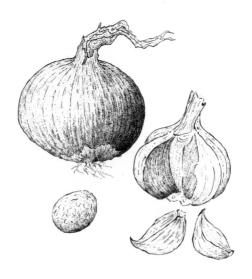

---

[6] For more information, see Stephen Barrett MD, 'Gastrointestinal Quackery: Colonics, Laxatives and More', revised 20 July 1999. Internet: Quackwatch Home Page.

7-DAY JUICING SLIMMING PLAN

This plan is based on easy-to-prepare meals totalling about 1,100 calories per day. It allows for an extra 150 ml/¼ pt/⅔ cup of semi-skimmed milk for tea and coffee, and thinly spread low-fat spreads.

DAY ONE

Fruit juice	No 10: Aloha Delight (see page 124)
Breakfast	2 weetabix with 150 ml/¼ pt/⅔ cup semi-skimmed milk
Snack	2 slices of wholemeal bread 25 g/1 oz lean ham, lettuce and tomato A few grapes
Vegetable juice	No 7: Weight Watcher's Wonder (see page 145)
Main meal	150 g/5 oz lean pork chop, grilled (broiled) 150 g/5 oz boiled new potatoes 75 g/3 oz leeks 30 ml/2 tbsp Hollandaise sauce (mayonnaise thinned down with skimmed milk and 5 ml/1 tsp lemon juice) 1 apple

DAY TWO

Fruit juice	No 17: Melon Medley (see page 128)
Breakfast	½ banana, sliced 1 shredded wheat 150 ml/5 fl oz semi-skimmed milk
Snack	50 g/2 oz hummus 1 wholemeal pitta bread 1 tomato and 1 apple
Vegetable juice	No 2: Winter's Tonic (see page 142)

Main meal	Chicken pasta salad made with:
	    50 g/2 oz wholewheat pasta twists
	    150 g/5 oz chicken breasts, cooked in a
	       little dry white wine
	    50 g/2 oz cooked broccoli spears
	    50 g/2 oz mushrooms, sliced
	    25 g/1 oz red (bell) pepper, seeded and
	       thinly sliced
	    1 spring onion (scallion), chopped
	75 g/3 oz low-fat ice cream

DAY THREE

Fruit juice	No 14: Morning Pick-up (see page 126)
Breakfast	1 poached or boiled egg A slice of wholemeal bread

Snack	150 g/5 oz jacket potato filled with
	    100 g/4 oz fromage frais or low-fat
	    cottage cheese
	A large raw salad, e.g. lettuce, spinach,
	    beansprouts, carrots, tomatoes, (bell)
	    peppers
	100 g/4 oz fresh fruit

Vegetable juice	No 9: The Body Builder (see page 146)

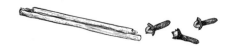

Main meal	175 g/6 oz steamed white fish
	175 g/6 oz boiled new potatoes
	75 g/3 oz broccoli or 2 carrots cut into julienne strips, steamed until just tender and devilled: fry (sauté) 2.5 ml/½ tsp paprika in 15 ml/1 tbsp vegetable oil to bring out the flavour, then add the carrot strips with 15 ml/1 tbsp lemon juice and stir until well coated
	30 ml/2 tbsp thin parsley sauce
	Two apricots stewed in orange juice

DAY FOUR

Fruit juice	No 2: Apple and Ginger Pear (see page 120)
Breakfast	30 g/1¼ oz sugar-free muesli topped with 150 g/5 oz freshly grated fruit and a 150 g/5 oz carton of plain yoghurt
Snack	1 sachet of low-calorie soup, made up as directed
	A granary roll with a thin scraping of low-fat spread
	50 g/2 oz half-fat Cheddar-type cheese and sliced tomatoes
	2 satsumas or 1 orange
Vegetable juice	No 14: Carrot and Apple Juice Lifesaver (see page 148)
Main meal	Lamb kebabs made with:
	100 g/4 oz lean lamb, cubed
	¼ green (bell) pepper, cut into squares
	4 button mushrooms
	4 cherry tomatoes
	15 ml/1 tbsp brown rice, cooked
	A green salad
	Onion sauce made with:
	1 onion, sliced
	150 ml/¼ pint/⅔ cup semi-skimmed milk
	10 ml/2 tsp cornflour (cornstarch)

DAY FIVE

Fruit juice	No 21: Tropical Cancer Fighter (see page 130)
Breakfast	25 g/1 oz porridge oats made with 200 ml/7 fl oz/scant 1 cup semi-skimmed milk with ½ banana, sliced, and 15 ml/1 tbsp raisins or l5 ml/1 tbsp clear honey
Snack	A granary bap with tomato and mozzarella salad 1 small low-fat yoghurt
Vegetable juice	No 10: Fennel, Beetroot and Apple Juice (see page 146)
Main meal	150 g/5 oz lean rump steak, grilled (broiled) 175 g/6 oz boiled new potatoes A green bean salad made with: Watercress ¼ green (bell) pepper ¼ red pepper ½ red onion, sliced 25 g/1 oz raw mushrooms, sliced 10 ml/2 tsp lemon juice 5 ml/1 tsp olive oil Fresh fruit or a slice of honeydew melon

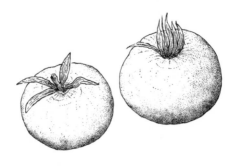

DAY SIX

Fruit juice	No 19: Aphrodite's Love Potion (see page 129)
Breakfast	A slice of wholemeal toast topped with 50 g/2 oz/¼ cup low-fat cottage cheese, 15 g/½ oz grated Cheddar cheese and a dash of Worcestershire sauce, lightly grilled (broiled)
Snack	2 slices of wholemeal bread 50 g/2 oz cooked white turkey or chicken meat with lettuce and tomato
Vegetable juice	No 20: The Garlic Stomach Cleanser (see page 151)
Main meal	Prawn and courgette gumbo: heat 15 ml/1 tsp olive oil, add the following ingredients and stir-fry until tender: 1 onion, chopped 1 garlic clove ½ green (bell) pepper, seeded and chopped 75 g/3 oz tinned tomatoes, chopped 75 g/3 oz courgette (zucchini), chopped 100 g/4 oz cooked peeled prawns (shrimp) Chopped parsley A pinch of dried thyme A pinch of cayenne pepper 75 g/3 oz cauliflower or broccoli A peach cooked in wine, served with a little low-fat yoghurt

DAY SEVEN

Fruit juice	No 6: Hawaiian Sunrise (see page 122)
Breakfast	2 rashers (slices) of very lean back bacon, grilled (broiled)
	2 tomatoes, grilled
	4 mushrooms, grilled
	A slice of wholemeal toast
	150 g/5 oz carton of plain or diet fruit yoghurt
Snack	75 g/3 oz sardines in tomato sauce, drained
	A slice of wholemeal toast
	A green salad, i.e. lettuce, (bell) peppers, endive, dressed with lemon juice
	Melon and strawberry salad
Vegetable juice	No 1: Italian Serenade (see page 141)
Main meal	150 g/5 oz roast chicken, lamb or beef
	1 jacket potato
	A medley of stir-fry vegetables and grated carrots seasoned and baked in 15 ml/ 1 tbsp water, 15 ml/1 tbsp lemon juice and a knob of butter in a low oven
	Baked banana in a liqueur, served with natural yoghurt

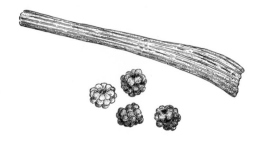

DICTIONARY OF JUICES

In future man will use the sunshine element of plants to regenerate and heal the human body.

George Crile MD

This list of fruit and vegetable juices has been compiled from a wide range of sources and briefly highlights their natural benefits, some of them based on folklore medicine. The responsive conditions mentioned are merely a guide to remedies and their therapeutic benefits to general health and, as I point out in the Dictionary of Conditions (see pages 83–94), the information given is NOT intended to replace medical advice: only a trained physician can diagnose and treat serious illness. All the juices listed, however, can provide you with healthy and enjoyable nourishment.

ALFALFA *Medicago sativa*
Alfalfa sprout mixes well with all vegetable juices and when combined with carrot and lettuce juice it is reputed to aid hair growth. It is a concentrated source of vitamin A. Its high vitamin K content is important as a blood clotting factor, and it also contains many valuable minerals. The best way to obtain alfalfa sprout for juicing is to grow your own from organic alfalfa seed (see page 79). Known as 'the king of sprouts', alfalfa is one of the most valuable plants on earth. Its roots can reach 12 m/ 40 ft into the subsoil, drawing up buried minerals.
    Dilute with carrot juice.

Responsive conditions
Anaemia, broken bones, eye disorders, fatigue, hair loss, impotence, kidney disorders, liver disorders, pregnancy and childbirth, sinusitis, thyroid gland regulation, weight loss

APPLE *Pyrus malus*
Fresh apple juice made from unpeeled apples is rich in vitamins and minerals, and a very high percentage of

vitamin A is concentrated in apple skins. The vitamin C content helps prevent colds, flu and intestinal infections and activates the body's elaborate defence system against bacterial toxins. The substantial amount of fruit pectin in fresh apple juice is responsible for its cloudiness. The pectin forms a gel in our intestines, absorbs and dissolves toxins, and stimulates peristalsis, the wave-like motion that moves food through the digestive tract. This can help to eliminate constipation or diarrhoea. Apple juice is rich in malic acid, which cleanses and heals inflammatory conditions. Storage may considerably reduce vitamin C levels.

Apple juice is the only fruit juice that can be mixed with any vegetable juice, and I find it very useful in all my juicing programmes.

Responsive conditions
Anaemia, arthritis, circulatory weakness, constipation, cystitis, gout, headache and migraine, indigestion, kidney disorders, liver disorders, rheumatism, weight loss

APRICOT *Prunus armeniaca*
Apricots contain much vitamin C. They also have a high concentration of beta-carotene especially in the ripened fruit, which may help the body prevent cancer. They contain potassium and magnesium, two minerals that supply us with energy, stamina and endurance, as well as iron for blood formation and silicon for healthy hair and skin. Apricots are high in malic acid, and are therefore beneficial for healing and cleansing.

Responsive conditions
Anaemia, cancer, constipation

ARTICHOKE, JERUSALEM *see* Jerusalem Artichoke

ASPARAGUS *Asparagus officinalis*
A good provider of vitamins A, C and E and folic acid, and the minerals potassium, magnesium and iron. The therapeutic properties of the juice exert a rapid effect upon the kidneys, acting as a good diuretic (you can also save asparagus cooking water for this purpose). It is a

purifier of the blood, tones up the nervous system and has gentle laxative properties.

Asparagus juice is usually taken three times a day in sherry-glass sized quantities, or mixed with carrot or celery juice.

Responsive conditions
Acne, anaemia, asthma, cancer, eye disorders, gout, kidney disorders, liver disorders, muscular disorders, nervous disorders, prostate disorders, rheumatism, skin disorders, varicose veins

BEANS *Phaseolus spp.*
(French (green), haricot (navy), runner, string)
A good source of vitamin A, present as its precursor beta-carotene, and a moderate source of vitamin C, iron, fibre and folate. Beans also contain substances that inhibit the formation of tumours.

Juice the stem, peel, leaves and seeds for ultimate nutrition. Mix half-and-half with carrot juice.

Responsive conditions
Anaemia, diabetes, fatigue, gout, hypoglycaemia, liver disorders, rheumatism, skin disorders

BEANSPROUT *Phaseolus spp.*
(i.e. various species can be used)
Lentils, aduki and mung beans make excellent sources of protein, and their juices mix well with other juices. They are an excellent source of vitamin C and iron. Avoid buying beansprouts that feel limp as they are not fresh.

Responsive conditions
Anaemia, arthritis, diabetes, digestive weakness, fatigue, fluid retention, muscular problems, weight loss

BEETROOT (RED BEET) *Beta vularis*
Beetroot and their dark green tops are very powerful cleansers and builders of the blood. The green shoots have a high quantity of chlorophyll and more iron than is found in spinach, and the whole vegetable is a good source of vitamins A (as beta-carotene), C and B6. Beetroot is a rich source of calcium, potassium, choline,

folate, organic sodium and natural sugars. After carrot, beetroot juice is one of the chief juices in the science of natural healing and is much used in convalescence on the continent.

The juice is potent and powerful, so use moderately. 50 g/2 oz of beetroot juice (from approximately ¼ beetroot) mixed with 175 g/6 oz of apple, carrot or cucumber juice is ample.

Responsive conditions
Anaemia, arthritis, bladder disorders, cancer, circulatory weakness, colitis, cystitis, depression, diarrhoea, eczema, eye fatigue, fatigue, heart disease, high blood pressure, jaundice, kidney disorders, liver disorders, laryngitis, menopause, menstrual problems, muscular problems, nervous disorders, prostate disorders, rheumatism, skin disorders, thrush, weight loss

BLACKBERRY *Rubus fruticosus*
An excellent source of vitamins A, C and E, iron, magnesium, calcium and fibre, and is high in carbohydrates. Their acids make them a valuable relief for diarrhoea and the iron is a good source for vegetarians.

Responsive conditions
Astringent, circulatory weakness, diarrhoea, menopause

BLACKCURRANT *Ribes spp.*
Blackcurrants are especially rich in vitamin C, a protection against cancer and heart disease. A substance in the fruit inhibits oxidation, giving the syrup a long shelf-life. It is unusual in that it contains three other nutrients not normally found in appreciable amounts in fruit – calcium, magnesium and vitamin E. The juice is also known as a good home remedy for sore throats.

Redcurrants and whitecurrants have less vitamin C. Unlike blackcurrants, whitecurrants contain high levels of potassium and calcium, but only trace amounts of vitamins A and E.

Responsive conditions
Circulatory weakness, convalescence, cystitis, respiratory problems

BLUEBERRY *Vaccinium spp.*

More commonly used in the USA than in Britain, blueberries provide carbohydrate energy. They are an excellent source of vitamin C, and a moderate source of iron and fibre. The acids in the fruit help prevent or control bladder problems. The juiced leaves are said to help reduce blood sugar for diabetics.

Responsive conditions
Acne, astringent, bladder disorders, canker sores, diarrhoea, protects blood vessel walls

BROCCOLI *Brassica oleracea*

Broccoli belongs to the cabbage family, and it is one of the vegetables that doctors now recommend as cancer fighters. A chemical, called sulforaphane, has been identified by Professor Paul Talalay and his colleagues at the Johns Hopkins University, USA, that has very definite anti-cancer properties, and this now makes broccoli a superstar vegetable. A good source of fibre, calcium and iron, with an abundance of vitamins A, C and E, and so an excellent food for vegetarians.

Juice it and mix with other vegetables, or stir-fry it.

Responsive conditions
Anxiety, cancer, circulatory weakness, cystitis, depression, fatigue, joint problems, motion sickness, nausea, stress, thrush

BRUSSELS SPROUTS *Brassica oleracea va. gemmifera*

Another member of the cabbage family that is an excellent source of vitamin C. It is a moderate source of fibre, phosphorus, iron and vitamin A (as beta-carotene). A combination of Brussels sprout, carrot and lettuce juice is said to improve the insulin-producing capacity of the pancreas, which should bring cheer to diabetics.

Responsive conditions
Acne, bladder disorders, blood pressure disorders, colitis, constipation, diabetes, digestive problems, fatigue, infection, kidney disorders, nervous disorders

CABBAGE *Brassica oleracea*

Cabbage, a member of the Brassica genus, is related to broccoli, Brussels sprouts, cauliflower, kale and kohlrabi. It is an excellent source of vitamin C, a good source of folate, and a moderate source of vitamin A (as beta-carotene). The outer leaves may contain 50 times as much beta-carotene as the inner white ones. Raw cabbage has a high level of vitamin C and folate, which makes it very beneficial in a juicing programme. It is said to be very good for stomach ulcers.

Mix it with other vegetables, especially carrot.

Responsive conditions

Asthma, bladder disorders, blood pressure disorders, bronchitis, circulatory weakness, colitis, constipation, fatigue, fever, hair loss, halitosis, kidney problems, mouth ulcers, pyorrhoea, skin disorders, stress, ulcers

CARROT *Daucus carota*

Carrot juice is very often referred to as 'the king of the vegetable juices'. It is very versatile; it can be mixed with all other vegetable juices, adding a sweet flavour, and it blends very well with apple juice. In fact, I juice three or four carrots and an apple every day as part of my juicing routine. Carrots have by far the highest beta-carotene level of any vegetable and beta-carotene is converted by the body into vitamin A (see Comparison Charts, page 178). Older, more mature carrots have the highest level of beta-carotene. In addition to their abundance of beta-carotene, carrots are a moderate source of vitamin C (though cooking greatly reduces the content), and contain some vitamins B, E and K, as well as the minerals calcium, phosphorus, potassium, sodium and other trace minerals. Eyes, skin, hair and nails all benefit from carrot juice. If you drink over 1.2 litres/2 pts/5 cups a day your skin can take on an orange glow, which does you no harm and will disappear as soon as you decrease your intake. Carrots have a tonic and cleansing effect on the liver, releasing stale bile and excess fats, and they therefore reduce cholesterol levels.

There are said to be 300 varieties of carrots in the world, with varying degrees of sweetness. The American

Californian carrot yields 350 g/12 oz/1½ cups of sugar from 1 litre/1¾ pts/4¼ cups of carrots juiced, and the English carrot yields only about 75 g/3 oz/⅓ cup, so you should expect variations in the amount of juice yielded by the carrots you buy. If picked straight from the garden, try and juice as much stem as possible as this part is loaded with vitamin K.

Responsive conditions
Acne, anxiety, arthritis, asthma, bladder problems, bone problems, cancer, cataracts, circulatory weakness, cystitis, depression, diabetes, diarrhoea, digestive weakness, eczema, eye disorders, gout, haemorrhoids, halitosis, hangover, kidney disorders, laryngitis, liver disorders, menopause, mouth ulcers, muscular weakness, nervous disorders, prostate disorders, rheumatism, sinusitis, skin disorders, stress, thrush, ulcers, varicose veins, weight loss

CAULIFLOWER *Brassica oleracea*
Cauliflower is available all year round. It is an excellent source of vitamin C and folate and provides a good source of potassium and phosphorous. It is best combined with carrot or apple juice, which makes it easier to digest. The outer leaves should be springy, never limp, for juicing.

Responsive condition
Fatigue

CELERY *Apium graveolens*
The organic sodium (salt) in celery makes this juice an excellent component of any vegetable combination. It has a calming effect on nervous conditions and is good for weight-reducing diets. The greener the stalks, the more nutritious they are. Beta-carotene is found in the green leaves, while vitamins C and E and the B-complex are in the stalks, which also contain calcium, potassium, sulphur, magnesium, iron and sodium. It is said that the sodium–potassium balance helps alleviate muscle cramping and fatigue. The combination of celery juice and apple juice is believed to relieve insomnia and to cleanse the body of excessive carbon dioxide, especially in polluted areas.

Responsive conditions
Anxiety, asthma, bronchitis, circulatory weakness, constipation, cystitis, diabetes, diarrhoea, eye disorders, fluid retention, gout, headache and migraine, insomnia, kidney disorders, liver disorders, mouth ulcers, muscular problems, nervous disorders, rheumatism, stress, weight loss

CHERRY *Prunus spp.*
Cherry juice contains beta-carotene and vitamin C, as well as calcium, chlorine, magnesium, phosphorous, sodium, sulphur, high potassium and trace elements of cobalt, copper, manganese and zinc. It is said to be helpful in cases of arthritis and gout.

Discard the stones (pits), using a cherry stoner, and mix with equal parts water or apple juice as the juice is quite strong.

Responsive conditions
Anaemia, arthritis, catarrh, constipation, cramps, gallstones, gout, indigestion, menstrual problems, prostate disorders, rheumatism, sciatica, weight loss

COURGETTE (ZUCCHINI) *Cucurbita pepo*
A rich source of vitamin C and, like cucumber, a refreshing thirst-quencher. It also acts as an internal body brush, cleansing the whole system. It's excellent mixed with carrot and garlic.

Responsive condition
Bladder disorders

CRANBERRY *Vaccinium macrocarpum*
Widely marketed in the United States, they usually arrive in Britain in time for the Christmas festivities. The juice contains vitamins A, B6 and C and folic acid. It also includes the minerals calcium, iron, phosphorus, potassium, sodium and sulphur. Cranberries are said to be very useful for urinary tract problems and a substance in the juice can provide temporary relief of lung congestion.

Responsive conditions
Asthma, bladder disorders, cystitis, diarrhoea, fever, fluid retention, indigestion, kidney disorders, lung disorders, prostate disorders, skin disorders, urinary tract infection, weight loss

CUCUMBER *Cacumis sativus*
Cucumbers are natural coolants. The juice is good for the complexion and may promote hair and fingernail growth and even prevent hair loss. The juice has an acceptable but unusual taste so always blend a small quantity, about 25–50 g/1–2 oz, with carrot juice. Cucumbers contain a great deal of water, and they help regulate the body temperature and are a natural diuretic. Vitamin A lies in the skin, but peel and discard the skin if waxed.

Responsive conditions
Acne, arthritis, bladder disorders, circulatory weakness, constipation, eczema, fatigue, fever, fluid retention, hair loss, halitosis, hangover, high blood pressure, kidney disorders, laryngitis, prostate disorders, rheumatism, scaly skin disorders (psoriasis), weight loss

CURLY KALE *see* Kale

DANDELION *Taraxacum officinale*
Dandelions have long been renowned as a herbal medicine with diuretic properties. They are exceptionally high in vitamins A and B1, in minerals and important trace elements. Along with the juices of the stinging nettle and watercress, dandelion juice is used for a bodily 'spring clean'. The treatment regulates the functioning of the gall bladder and has a beneficial effect on the nervous system. It is also said to give firmness to the teeth and gums and prevent tooth decay. Like carrot juice it is said to improve eyesight and prevent night blindness.

The juice tastes slightly bitter so use only 50 g/2 oz at a time, blended with sweeter-tasting juices such as carrot or apple.

Responsive conditions
Acne, anaemia, bladder disorders, bone disorders, circulatory weakness, constipation, depression, eye disorders, headache and migraine, heart problems, kidney disorders, liver disorders, nervous disorders, skin disorders, thrush, weight loss

DRIED FRUITS *see* Prunes and Dried Fruits

ELDERBERRY *Sambus nigra*
The elderberry grows wild throughout Europe and has a history of medicinal applications. It is important to choose only very ripe berries, as the unripe fruit contains poisonous alkaloids. Elderberries are a good source of vitamin A and a moderate source of vitamin C, which assists in the prevention of colds. The juice can soothe the chest and induces sweating, which is thought to be beneficial in a feverish cold. It is a mild laxative and has diuretic properties.

Responsive conditions
Colds, constipation, fluid retention, respiratory infection

ENDIVE *Cichorium spp.*
A salad leaf vegetable in a rosette of green curly leaves. It has a food element constantly needed by the optic system and, combined with carrot, celery and parsley, it refurnishes the optic nerve and muscular system and is one of the richest sources of vitamin A among green vegetables.

Responsive conditions
Anaemia, bladder disorders, constipation, eye disorders, gall bladder problems, heart problems, liver disorders, skin disorders, weight loss

FENNEL *Foeniculum vulgare*

Fennel is a versatile vegetable and the bulb and leaves have a liquorice flavour. A relative of celery, it contains an essential oil soothing to an irritated stomach. It is similar to celery in nutrients, but lower in sodium, and high in energy-giving sugars. The juice is especially helpful in relaxing and calming the nerves.

Mix the juice with other green sprouts and vegetable juices, which will give it a pleasant flavour and aroma. It's also delicious mixed with apple juice.

Responsive conditions
Arthritis, bronchitis, gout, headache and migraine, kidney disorders, liver disorders, menstrual problems, nervous disorders, skin disorders, weight loss

FENUGREEK *Trigonella goenum-graecum*

A leguminous plant related to clover, grown in classical times for the medicinal properties of its seeds. The sprouted leaves are used as a salad vegetable, or cooked like spinach. It has pleasant, slightly bitter taste. Mix with apple or carrot juice.

Responsive conditions
Fluid retention, heart problems, skin disorders, weight loss

GARLIC *Allium sativum*

Garlic is a powerful healer and an important anti-oxidant. Evidence has suggested that garlic reduces blood pressure, lowers the incidence of blood clotting, prevents stomach cancer and boosts the immune system. The component in garlic called allicun, which gives it the smell, is thought likely to inhibit bacterial growth and destroy fungi and yeast in the body and rid the body of toxins through the skin. Garlic is high in potassium, iron, iodine and phosphorus.

To prevent odours lingering in the machine, juice one or two cloves first, followed by carrots, a little parsley, celery, beetroot (red beet) or apples. Alternatively, crush them separately and add to the juiced vegetables.

Responsive conditions
Anxiety, asthma, blood pressure disorders, cancer, circulatory weakness, depression, fatigue, fever, headache and migraine, joint disorders, respiratory disorders, sinusitis, skin disorders, stress, thrush, urinary tract disorders

GRAPE *Vitis vinifera*
Grape juice contains supplies of vitamins A, Bl, B2 and a little C, niacin and an abundance of minerals. It is a good source of tartaric acid and energy-producing sugar. Grapes stimulate kidney function and help regulate the heartbeat; they cleanse the liver and eliminate uric acid from the body; they soothe the nervous system. Grape juice is easily digested.

Responsive conditions
Anaemia, anxiety, blood disorders, cancer, catarrh, constipation, fever, gout, haemorrhoids, indigestion, kidney disorders, liver disorders, menstrual problems, rheumatism, skin disorders, stress, tumours, weight loss

GRAPEFRUIT *Citris paradisi*
Grapefruit juice is rich in vitamin C and in the minerals calcium, phosphorous and potassium, and contains lesser amounts of various other minerals. The high content of bioflavonoids in the white pulp helps the body to retain and use vitamin C, so when juicing leave as much pith on the fruit as you can and only discard the outer peel. Pink grapefruits are very high in beta-carotene – 280 ug per l00 g/4 oz.

Responsive conditions
Bruises, cancer, catarrh, colds, coughs, ear disorders, fatigue, fever, gout, hangover, indigestion, insomnia, liver disorders, menopause, pregnancy, pyorrhoea, scurvy and other skin disorders, sore throat, varicose veins, weight loss

HORSERADISH *Armoracia rusticana*

Horseradish contains an efficient solvent of mucus or phlegm in the system. The ground root, which has a sharp, burning flavour, must be taken in quantities of not more than 2.5 ml/½ tsp at a time because, while it stimulates the appetite and aids in the secretion of digestive juices, large amounts can irritate the kidneys and bladder.

Responsive condition
Coughs

JERUSALEM ARTICHOKE *Helianthus tuberosus*

The Jerusalem artichoke makes a useful juice for diabetics as it is loaded with natural inulin (not insulin), an energy source similar to sugar. A small, gnarled tuberous vegetable, it is an excellent source of non-starchy carbohydrates and it is said to reduce a craving for sweets. It is a very good source of potassium.

50 g/2 oz of Jerusalem artichoke juice to 175–225 g/ 6–8 oz of other vegetable juices, such as carrot, makes a palatable drink.

Responsive conditions
Diabetes, fatigue, hypoglycaemia, weight loss

KALE *Brassica oleracea*

A member of the cabbage family with an exceptionally high calcium, chlorophyll and vitamins A (beta-carotene) C and E content and they are packed with blood-building iron. The juice is especially beneficial to the eyesight, bones, teeth, blood and lymph glands, which swell if they are calcium deficient.

It has a strong taste, so is best blended with other vegetable juices or apple juice.

Responsive conditions
Anaemia, anxiety, arthritis, asthma, cancer, circulatory weakness, cystitis, depression, diabetes, eye disorders, fatigue, hair loss, hangover, hay fever, impotence, liver disorders, motion sickness, muscular problems, nausea, pregnancy and childbirth, pyorrhoea, skin disorders, stress, thrush, ulcers, weight loss

KIWI FRUIT (CHINESE GOOSEBERRY)
Actinidia chinensis

A popular fruit worldwide, native to China but large quantities are now grown in New Zealand, California and Israel. Kiwi fruit are very rich in nutrients and they have twice as much vitamin C as oranges. They are rich in potassium too, vital to every cell in our body, a deficiency of which can lead to high blood pressure, depression, fatigue and poor digestion.

Responsive conditions

Catarrh, circulatory weakness, colds and flu, coughs, digestive weakness, fatigue, high blood pressure, skin disorders, sore throat, stress, weight loss

KOHLRABI *Brassica oleracea varr. gongyloides*

Kohlrabi resembles a turnip, except that it grows above ground so it is a swollen stem not a root. It is an excellent source of vitamin C, carbohydrates and chlorophyll and minerals such as calcium, potassium and iron.

Mix it with other green juices.

Responsive conditions

Asthma, catarrh, eczema, lung disorders, sinus disorders, skin disorders, thyroid disorders, weight loss

LEEK *Allium ampeloprasum varr. porrum*

The Egyptians, Greeks and Romans prized leeks for their medicinal value. They have much the same healing properties as onions and garlic and act as an internal antiseptic. They are an excellent source of vitamins A and C, iron and most minerals.

Responsive conditions

Arthritis, constipation, joint disorders, respiratory disorders, urinary tract disorders

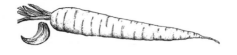

LEMON *Citrus limon*
Lemons have more vitamin C than oranges as well as B vitamins. Lemon juice protects the mucous membranes lining the digestive tract. Lemon peel contains a substance that helps the body absorb vitamin C, so juice the entire fruit.

Dilute the juice with water and drink it before breakfast to keep your bowels regular.

Responsive conditions
Anaemia, asthma, blood disorders, cancer, catarrh, colds, constipation, coughs, cystitis, ear disorders, fever, gout, hangover, indigestion, infection, liver disorders, pneumonia, pyorrhoea, rheumatism, scurvy and other skin disorders, sore throat, weight loss

LETTUCE *Lactuca sativa*
There are many and various types of lettuce. The deep green lettuce is an excellent source of calcium, chlorophyll, iron, magnesium, potassium, silicon, and vitamins A and E and some C. Lettuce juice adds shine, thickness and health to the hair and improves the skin. The iceberg lettuce is said to calm the nerves and relax the muscles.

Mix the juice with other green, sprout and vegetable juices.

Responsive conditions
Acne, anaemia, constipation, diabetes, hair loss, insomnia, liver disorders, motion sickness, muscular problems, nausea, nervous disorders, prostate disorders, weight loss

LIME *Citrus aurantifolia*
Similar to lemon juice and with the same benefits, but not as acidic and a good body cleanser.

Responsive conditions
Anaemia, blood disorders, cancer, colds and flu, constipation, coughs, ear disorders, fever, gout, hair loss, hangover, infection, insomnia, liver disorders, nervous disorders, pneumonia, pyrrohoea, sore throat, weight loss

MANGO *Mangifera indica*

The 'king of tropical fruits', it has very high levels of vitamin A (beta-carotene), moderate amounts of iron, and one medium-sized mango provides the recommended daily intake of vitamin C. It also has high levels of magnesium, calcium, potassium and phosphorus. They vary very much in size.

This is a fruit I prefer to eat whole, but for juicing you should halve the fruit horizontally, remove the large stone (pit), then strip off the tough outer skin.

Responsive conditions
Acne, constipation, hangover, indigestion, kidney disorders, liver disorders, ulcers, weight loss

MELON *Cucumis melo*

There are many types of melon – honeydew, casaba, charentais, ogen, santa claus, Spanish, cantaloupe and watermelon, to name but a few.[7] They are all rich in vitamins A and C and the B-complex vitamins, which makes them good skin and nerve food. They all have a variety of minerals, enzymes and plenty of natural unconcentrated sugar. They are cooling and have a tonic effect on digestion.

Juice the entire melon and always eat or drink it by itself.

Responsive conditions
Anxiety, arthritis, bladder disorders, constipation, cramps, cystitis, fluid retention, headache and migraine, kidney disorders, mouth ulcers, prostate disorders, skin disorders, stress, varicose veins, weight loss

NETTLES *Urtica dioica et urens*

Nettle juice has been used for centuries in natural healing. The herbalist Thomas Culpeper said 'the juice is a safe and sure medicine to open the pipes and passages of the

---

[7] In America, the Center for Science in the Public Interest listed fruits by nutrient value. The cantaloupe melon topped the list, closely followed by watermelons, then oranges, strawberries, grapefruit, pineapples, tangerines and peaches. Plums came towards the end.

lungs'. Nettles are rich in minerals, especially iron, and in folk medicine they are strongly recommended for their tonic and blood purifying powers. In small amounts nettle juice is thought to be useful in healing haemorrhoids (piles).

Use only the first five leaves of young nettles in the spring – the autumn leaves are unwholesome. The treatment for haemorrhoids is 15 ml/1 tbsp nettle juice three times a day. Dilute with carrot juice to make it more palatable.

Responsive conditions
Anaemia, bladder disorders, bleeding gums, eczema, haemorrhoids, kidney disorders, nervous disorders

ONION *Allium cepa*
Along with garlic, the onion enjoys a high reputation for its curative properties. The Greeks and Romans used the juice for all digestive problems and as a blood purifier. Onions are a good source of vitamin C and contain more sugar than many other vegetables. They are rich in copper and iron as well as sulphur, calcium, phosphorus, potassium and iodine.

The juice is strong, so mix it in small amounts with other vegetable juices.

Responsive conditions
Bladder disorders, catarrh, circulatory weakness, coughs, digestive disorders, fatigue, fever, heart disease, respiratory disorders, skin disorders, weight loss

ORANGE *Citrus sinensis*
Compared with other fruits the orange is very nutritious, and the freshly squeezed fruit or peeled and juiced whole fruit is far superior in taste and nutrients to bottled or frozen orange juice. The juice is rich in vitamin A, contains some vitamin C and small amounts of vitamins B1, B2, B6, E and K, biotin, folic acid, inositol, niacin, bioflavonoids and 11 amino acids. There are also many minerals in oranges. Along with grapefruit and lemon juices, orange juice cleanses and tones the gastrointestinal tract. The heart and lungs also benefit, and overly acidic

blood is alkalised by drinking orange juice on a regular basis (four doses of about 175 g/6 oz a week). Blood oranges are much higher in beta-carotene, a vitamin A precursor.

To juice, remove the skin thinly but leave as much of the white pith and membrane on the fruit as possible as this is beneficial and helps the system to absorb the vitamin C.

Responsive conditions
Anaemia, asthma, blood disorders, cancer, catarrh, colds, coughs, fatigue, fever, gout, hangover, heart disease, high blood pressure, indigestion, liver disorders, lung disorders, menopause, pneumonia, pyorrhoea, rheumatism, scurvy and other skin disorders, sore throat, weight loss

PAPAYA *Carica papaya*
This tropical fruit (which should not be confused with the papaw fruit from a small North American tree) has a fine-tasting juice. It's very high in vitamins A and C. It also supplies iron and is a boon to weightwatchers as it has no sucrose but contains laevulose, which is especially suitable for diabetics. It contains an active principal called *papain*, which has long been recognised as being of considerable value in dyspepsia and helps to digest protein. Papain is used commercially to tenderise meat.

Discard the seeds before juicing (they are used as a vermifuge treatment to expel intestinal worms in veterinary medicine) and peel the fruit before juicing. The rather thick juice can be thinned with water or it tastes very good with apple juice. They are also very good not juiced but eaten whole with a little lemon juice.

Responsive conditions
Acidosis, acne, blood disorders, colds and flu, constipation, coughs, diabetes, eczema, gout, heart disease, indigestion, kidney disorders, liver disorders, sciatica, sore throat, tumours, ulcers, weight loss

PARSLEY *Carum petroselinum – Petroselinum sativum*

A leading organic remedy, parsley is valued for its high content of chlorophyll, vitamins A, C and E, and minerals such as calcium, magnesium, phosphorus, potassium, sodium, sulphur and, especially, iron. It is a fine blood and body cleanser, particularly of the kidneys, liver and urinary tract. It is an aid to good eyesight.

The juice is very concentrated so must be mixed with other vegetable juices or apple juice. 25 g/1 oz mixed with 200 g/7 oz of another juice is recommended.

Responsive conditions
Anaemia, anxiety, arthritis, asthma, bladder disorders, cancer, circulatory weakness, cystitis, depression, diabetes, diarrhoea, eye disorders, fatigue, gout, headache and migraine, heart disease, kidney disorders, liver disorders, menopause, prostate disorders, skin disorders, stress, thrush, urinary tract infection, weight loss

PARSNIP *Pastinaca sativa*

The Elizabethans used parsnips as a sweetmeat with honey and spices, as well as serving it as a root vegetable. Parsnips are sweeter than carrots; three-quarters of the sugar in parsnips is in the form of sucrose which, when consumed in its natural form, is not damaging to the health. Parsnips are a good source of vitamin C, some E, chlorine, phosphorous, potassium, silicon and sulphur, so they are good for the nutrition of the skin, hair and nails.

Parsnip juice has a strong flavour, so it should be diluted with other vegetable juices or apple juice.

Responsive conditions
Acne, arthritis, asthma, bladder disorders, bone problems, cancer, cataract, diabetes, digestive weakness, eye disorders, hay fever, liver disorders, muscular weakness, pregnancy and childbirth, sinusitis, skin disorders, ulcers, weight loss

PAW PAW *see Papaya*

PEACH *Prunus persica*

Peaches are rich in vitamins A (beta-carotene), B-complex and C, as well as minerals such as calcium, potassium, manganese, chlorine and sulphur. The juice cleanses the intestines and stimulates activity in the lower bowl. It is also said to be helpful in the prevention of morning sickness.

Most of the nutritional value lies in the skin, so remove the stone (pit) and juice the whole peach. The juice is fairly thick so it can be mixed with water, apple or grape juice.

Responsive conditions
Blood disorders, constipation, indigestion, pregnancy

PEAR *Pyrus communis*

Pears are a good source of carbohydrate, fibre and folic acid. They contain vitamins A, B1, B2 and C and niacin. They are also rich in phosphorus and potassium and contain lesser amounts of other minerals. Like apples, pears are an important source of pectin, a valued aid to digestion, and they cleanse the body of toxins and other waste by stimulating bowel activity.

Buy firm but ripe pears for juicing. Pear juice mixes well with apple juice or can be diluted with water or lemon juice.

Responsive conditions
Bladder disorders, constipation, liver disorders, prostate disorders

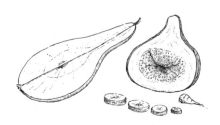

PEPPERS (BELL PEPPERS) OR CAPSICUMS
Capsicum annum
The difference between sweet green and sweet red peppers is age – the red pepper is simply a ripe green pepper. Fruits and vegetables with shiny skins are high in potassium and silicon: these nutrients certainly give the skin a healthy glow, and all varieties are beneficial to the hair and nails. They are a good source of vitamin C and a fully ripe red pepper is rich in vitamin A (beta-carotene). They also stimulate the circulation and tone and cleanse the arteries and heart muscles.

Dilute with other vegetable juices.

Responsive conditions
Acne, anxiety, arthritis, circulatory weakness, cystitis, depression, eye disorders, hair loss, heart disease, high blood pressure, motion sickness, muscular problems, nausea, skin disorders, stress

PINEAPPLE *Ananas comosus*
Pineapples contain bromelin, a very special enzyme that helps to balance and neutralise fluids that are either too alkaline or too acidic, and also stimulates hormonal secretion in the pancreas. Pineapples are loaded with minerals and vitamins A, B-complex and C. Because of the vitamin C content, pineapple is also very effective in soothing throats.

Choose pineapples with a yellow skin, that smell strong and sweet, and give a little when pressed. The thick skin contains many nutrients, so juice the entire fruit, if your juicer is powerful enough.

Responsive conditions
Acidosis, anxiety, blood disorders, colds, depression, gout, hangover, indigestion, kidney disorders, menopause, menstrual problems, pneumonia, pyorrhoea, sciatica, sore throat, stress, weight loss

PLUM *Prunus domestica*
Plums are related to peaches and some cherries and have to be stoned (pitted) for juicing. They provide vitamins A, C and E and iron, potassium, calcium and magnesium, as

well as carbohydrates for energy. They are high in malic acid, so are good for cleansing and healing.

Dilute thick plum juice with water or apple or grape juice.

Responsive conditions
Bladder disorders, circulatory weakness, constipation, fatigue

POMEGRANATE *Punca granatum*
The fruit is nearly 77 per cent water. It is very rich in sodium and vitamins B and C and also contains some vitamin A. It has a cleansing and cooling effect on the system and can act as a laxative.

Responsive conditions
Constipation, cystitis, menopause

POTATO *Solanum tuberosum*
In winter the potato is one of the most useful sources of vitamin C, though this content is reduced by 25 per cent when potatoes are cooked in their skins and by 50 per cent when peeled and diced. The peel is loaded with potassium, which is recommended for high blood pressure. In addition to vitamin C and potassium, they also contain vitamins A and B, sodium, calcium, magnesium, phosphorus, iron, manganese, copper and sulphur. Potato juice is very soothing on the digestive tract, so it is useful for gastric ulcers and arthritis. It relieves constipation and helps haemorrhoids. Used externally it is well known for cleansing skin blemishes.

Choose potatoes with eyes, which indicates that they are capable of sprouting, as they will be full of enzymes, and avoid potatoes with green-tinted skins. Raw potato juice is unpalatable and must be sweetened with honey or diluted with carrot, lemon or apple juice. Or it can be added to soups made by the juicer as a thickening agent instead of flour (only ¼ of a peeled potato is needed to thicken 600 ml/1 pt/2½ cups of soup).

Responsive conditions
Arthritis, circulatory weakness, constipation, digestive disorders, eczema, fatigue, haemorrhoids, muscular problems, peptic ulcers, varicose veins

PRUNES AND DRIED FRUITS *Prunus domestica*

Prune juice is a good source of vitamin A and the minerals copper and iron. There is benzoic and quinic acid present, which makes an excellent laxative. Plums are high in potassium, but show only traces of vitamin C.

You need a blender and a strainer to juice prunes and all dried fruits, not a home juicer. Soak 15 stoned (pitted) prunes overnight in 1.2 litres/2 pts/5 cups of hot water, then blend in the soaking water. Strain the juice and discard the pulp.

Responsive conditions
Anaemia, arthritis, constipation, haemorrhoids, weight loss

PURSLANE *Portulaca loeracea*

Purslane is widely used as a salad plant and is also cooked like spinach in the Far East.

Responsive conditions
Anaemia, bladder disorders, constipation, heart problems, skin disorders

QUINCE *cydonia oblonga*

An excellent source of vitamin C. The quinine extracted from quince has an anti-malarial action. It can be used only when tree-ripened, when the natural fruit sugars have matured. It has a sour taste, so mix small quantities of quince juice with apple or carrot juice.

Responsive condition
Constipation

RADISH *Raphanus sativus*

An excellent source of vitamin C, iron, magnesium and potassium. The juice stimulates the appetite and has an antiseptic effect in the intestinal tract. It is good for liver and gall bladder problems, is a blood cleanser and soothes the mucous membranes.

Use the green stems as well in juicing: they are very high in minerals as well as vitamins A (beta-carotene) and C. Used only a small handful at a time and mix well with other vegetable juices.

Responsive conditions
Arthritis, asthma, catarrh, eczema, liver disorders, lung disorders, sinusitis, skin problems, thrush, thyroid disorders, weight loss

RASPBERRY *Rubus idaeus*
Raspberries contain a significant amount of vitamin C, are high in iron, and have a moderate amount of magnesium, calcium, and potassium. Valued by herbalists for their cooling effect, they are also thought to be a useful aid in convalescence. According to Mrs Beeton, the nineteenth-century writer on household management, 'The berry itself is exceedingly wholesome, and invaluable to people of a nervous or bilious temperament.'

Raspberry juice can be diluted with apple juice: I like it with carrot juice sometimes (a rare exception to the fruit and vegetable mixing rule).

Responsive conditions
Circulatory weakness, convalescence, digestive disorders, nervous tension

RED SWISS CHARD *see* Swiss chard

REDCURRANT *see* Blackcurrant

ROOT GINGER *Zingiber officinale*
A thick tuberous rhizome which the Romans used for medicinal purposes. A juiced 1.5–2.5 cm/¼–½ in piece of the root gives a delicious zip to many fruit and vegetable cocktails. It is a good treatment for fever and has been recommended as an aid in healing vocal chords and as an expectorant to rid the sinus cavities of mucus and the lungs of phlegm.

Responsive conditions
Anxiety, fatigue, fever, headache and migraine, motion sickness, mouth ulcers, nausea, sinusitis, stress, thrush

SPINACH *Spinacea oleracea*

Spinach juice has a very important role to play in building the blood and revitalising the constitution. The juice is an excellent source of chlorophyll and a good source of vitamins A, B-complex and E, calcium, iron, magnesium, phosphorous, potassium, sodium and trace elements. It is rich in oxalic acid. It is said to have more protein than any other leafy vegetable, apart from seaweed. The juice strengthens the teeth and gums and has a mild laxative effect.

Spinach juice is best used in moderation (i.e. 30 ml/ 2 tbsp) mixed with a combination of other vegetables, preferably carrot, only once or twice a week.

Responsive conditions
Acne, anaemia, anxiety, arthritis, asthma, cancer, circulatory weakness, colitis, constipation, cystitis, depression, diabetes, diarrhoea, digestive weakness, eczema, eye disorders, fatigue, gout, haemorrhoids, hair loss, halitosis, heart problems, high blood pressure, infection, kidney disorders, laryngitis, liver disorders, menopause, motion sickness, mouth ulcers, muscular problems, nausea, nervous disorders, prostate disorders, pyorrhoea, skin disorders, stress, thrush, thyroid irregularity, ulcers, varicose veins, weight loss

SPRING GREENS (COLLARD GREENS)
Brassica oleracea, var. capitata

These are the first spring greens of a cabbage that grow before a head is formed, and they are good for juicing. Raw cabbage is an excellent source of vitamin C and folate. It also contains some beta-carotene, depending on the amount of chlorophyll, and the outer leaves may contain 50 times as much as the inner white leaves.

Responsive conditions
Asthma, bladder disorders, blood pressure disorders, bronchitis, circulatory weakness, colitis, constipation, fatigue, fever, hair loss, halitosis, kidney problems, mouth ulcers, pyorrhoea, skin disorders, stress, ulcers.

STRAWBERRY *Fragaria virginiana f.chiloensis*

All berry fruits are good for us, but strawberries are the best and home-grown ones the very best and generally considered better tasting. They are high in vitamin C, are a good source of folic acid, and have moderate amounts of iron. Ellagic acid is present, which reduces and neutralises the damaging effects of the carcinogen PAH found in cigarette smoke. This is just as important for non-smokers, as breathing secondhand smoke is thought to be as harmful as smoking itself. Strawberry juice is also highly cleansing to the blood, tissues and muscles.

Wash strawberries thoroughly, and remove the green stalks just before juicing. They make a strong, thick juice and may be mixed with apple juice, citrus fruit juices or water.

Responsive conditions

Acne, anxiety, constipation, fever, fluid retention, gout, indigestion, kidney disorders, menopause, motion sickness, nausea, pain, pneumonia, prostate disorders, pyorrhoea, rheumatism, stress, thyroid disease, weight loss

SWISS CHARD *Beta vulgaris spp. cicla*

Related to sugar beet and first grown in Sicily. It is grown for its green leaves, not the root, which taste like spinach. It is a good source of iron and pro-vitamin A and vitamin C. It must be mixed with other juices.

Responsive conditions

Anaemia, anxiety, asthma, bronchitis, cancer, fatigue, menopause, menstrual problems, muscular problems, skin disorders, thrush

TOMATO *Lycopersucon esculentum*

Tomatoes, sometimes known as love apples, are classed as a fruit, and they provide an excellent amount of vitamins A, C and E. They are a good source of potassium and there are trace elements of iron and iodine. Fresh, ripe home-grown tomatoes are best for juicing, and a mixture of carrot, spinach and tomato juices is very good for anaemic conditions – a popular way to serve it to children, who may need extra iron. Fresh tomato juice is said to be highly cleansing to the liver, and good for digestive upsets.

Responsive conditions
Anaemia, bladder disorders, digestive weakness, gout, kidney disorders, liver disorders, menopause, skin disorders, weight loss

TURNIP *Brassica rapa*
Turnip greens contain a massive amount of calcium, iron and vitamin A (beta-carotene), so chop them for juicing with the root, which contains potassium, calcium, phosphorous, magnesium, sulphur, copper, and vitamins A, B-complex and C. Turnip juice is said to make a good pick-me-up when you're run down or depressed. Some have reported it as being good for kidney stones.

Responsive conditions
Acne, anaemia, arthritis, asthma, bladder disorders, bronchitis, cancer, circulatory weakness, diabetes, eye disorders, fatigue, haemorrhoids, heart disease, infection, kidney disorders, liver disorders, lung disorders, motion sickness, nausea, skin disorders, thrush, varicose veins, weight loss

WATERCRESS *Nasturtium officinale*
Watercress is abundant in minerals, especially iron and calcium, and is an excellent source of vitamins A and C. It has great restorative powers as a purifier and strengthener of the blood, and holds a very special place in raw juice therapy. It also contains gluconasturtin, which when chewed, chopped or juiced neutralises a carcinogen in tobacco.

The juice is too strong to be taken neat, but its pleasant peppery flavour mixes well with carrot and other vegetable juices. Combined with cucumber and beetroot (red beet) juices it is said to remove the uric acid in some forms of rheumatism. Mixed with carrot, parsley and potato juices, it is believed to be helpful in clearing the lungs. Respiratory and urinary tract infections are said to benefit from doses of watercress juice.

Responsive Conditions
Acne, anaemia, asthma, bladder disorders, circulatory weakness, eczema, haemorrhoids, hair loss, intestinal disorders, kidney disorders, liver disorders, lung disorders, menstrual problems, muscular problems, respiratory problems, rheumatism, skin disorders, thyroid irregularity, urinary tract disorders, varicose veins, weight loss

WATERMELON *see Melon*

WHEATGRASS *Triticum*
Wheatgrass is commonly used in the United States. It is an excellent source of chlorophyll and is said to have the widest range of vitamins and minerals of any of the vegetables. It is believed to have remarkable regenerative and anti-ageing properties, and is highly recommended in America for cancer patients. Research by the English nutritionist Jackie Norton confirms that, because of its high level of antioxident enzymes, wheatgrass can help to alleviate toxic conditions. It can be grown at home on trays.

Responsive conditions
Acne, anaemia, anxiety, arthritis, asthma, bladder disorders, bone disorders, bronchitis, cancer, circulatory weakness, colitis, constipation, cystitis, diabetes, eye disorders, fatigue, hair loss, hay fever, heart disease, high blood pressure, hypoglycaemia, impotence, infection, kidney disorders, liver disorders, low blood pressure, mouth ulcers, nervous disorders, premature ageing, skin disorders, stress, ulcers, weight loss

WHITECURRANT *see Blackcurrant*

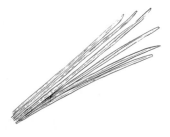

WHEATGRASS, SPROUTING AND APPLE JUICE

WHEATGRASS

Walk into any of the new health juicing bars springing up all over Britain, and you will see a tray of freshly grown, deep emerald green wheatgrass waiting to be juiced into 15 g/1 oz quantities, which can be taken alone or mixed with apple or carrot juice or a little mineral water.

The late Ann Wigmore, one of the founders of the Hippocrates Health Institute in Boston over 40 years ago, was one of the first to apply the benefits of wheatgrass juice to human health. A young woman at that time, she was suffering from an incurable disease but, by introducing wheatgrass juice to her diet on a daily basis, she managed to cure herself and she remained the epitome of health and vitality well into her eighties. Over those years she became recognised in the field of living foods nutrition for her research into the field of living foods nutrition and became a pioneer in research into the benefits of wheatgrass juice. She witnessed the complete reversal of many of the clinic's guests' symptoms who followed her wheatgrass and live foods diet. Although some of her claims were later found to be overenthusiastic and not fully scientifically based, the empirical evidence to support the health benefits of wheatgrass remains undeniable.

Her *The Wheatgrass Book*, published in 1985, cites international medical researches which she said backed her claim that, whether you suffer from chronic fatigue, sinusitis, ulcers or a more serious illness such as cancer, wheatgrass chlorophyll extracted from seven-day-old wheat sprouts can help you where even other medicines have failed – alongside, of course, a sound diet, exercise and a positive attitude to gaining good health. She stated that wheatgrass juice duplicates the molecular structure of haemoglobin, a vital part of the blood, and thought that, because it is so rich in free-radical scavengers (provided by its high incidence of provitamin A), it might inhibit malignancies (see The Cancer Story and Your Diet, pages 95–108). She said that the high chlorophyll in wheatgrass contains a cell stimulator and rejuvenator and red blood cell builder that purifies the blood, which helps to cleanse the kidneys, liver and urinary tract and therefore contributes to regularity and a healthy bowel.

THE CHLOROPHYLL IN WHEATGRASS

Thomas Edison once said: 'Until man duplicates a blade of grass, Nature can laugh at his so called scientific knowledge.'

The green juice of grasses has been valued since Biblical times, and for some time scientists have known about the deodorising properties of chlorophyll. That is why it is used in some drugs, toothpastes, chewing gum, breath fresheners, vaginal douches and antiseptics. The antibacterial compounds in wheatgrass juice, high in chlorophyll, are especially good at destroying the anaerobic bacteria that thrive in oxygen-poor blood and tissue. It deactivates the bacteria and promotes regeneration of the damaged area. Ann Wigmore referred to the rich supply of chlorophyll in wheatgrass juice as 'condensed solar energy', and said: 'Chlorophyll can protect us from carcinogens like no other food or medicine can. It acts to strengthen the cells, detoxify the liver and bloodstream, and chemically neutralise the polluting elements themselves.' In The Cancer Story and Your Diet, I refer to the use of wheatgrass juice in cancer treatments in medical research and more of the work of Ann Wigmore.

Wheatgrass juice is also said to contain anti-ageing properties and in recent years there has been much research conducted on this topic. Working independently at the London University and at the University of Cologne in Germany, scientists have found among those contributing components are: super oxide dismutase (SOD); vitamins A, B-complex, C and E; chlorophyll; a full spectrum of minerals and trace elements including calcium, iron, magnesium and potassium; a number of special enzymes; and amino acids (proteins).

Another, less understood, ingredient is called 'the grass juice factor'. Scientists working on animal nutrition confirm that a mixture of young cereal grasses fed to livestock improved milk production in cows and produced stronger, more resilient, longer-living animals, including guinea pigs, rats, rabbits, cats and ferrets. Further research revealed that grass feeds contain natural plant steroid hormones, which enhance fertility and improves lactation not only in many animals but also in humans. Research by the US Army has shown that chlorophyll-rich foods may be effective in decreasing the effects of radiation.

Wheatgrass juice is said to benefit the blood cells, bones, glands, hair, muscles, spleen, teeth and other body parts. It has been administered directly to the skin and scalp and implanted rectally to cleanse and heal the large intestine and has even been used to wash the eyes, gums, sinuses and teeth. It is also believed to protect the lungs and blood from air and water pollution, cigarette smoke, toxins and heavy metals. It is further said to be a safe and extremely effective aid to weight loss, as it suppresses the appetite and stimulates metabolism and circulation.

Humans do not have the ability to digest grass, so it must be juiced. Once juiced it will go off quickly, so it must be consumed within 15 minutes and it is best consumed on an empty stomach. Some experience nausea when they begin taking wheatgrass juice: if this occurs, reduce your intake and build gradually from 25 g/1 oz to 100 g/4 oz a day. It can, of course, be diluted with mineral water, carrot or apple juice.

HOW TO GROW WHEATGRASS

Although wheatgrass juice powder can be obtained from some health food stores it is very expensive, and there is nothing to beat harvesting your own wheatgrass for the ultimate juice nutrition.

You will need wheatgrass seeds, known in the UK as wheatgrain, which can be obtained from your local health food store. You can use other grains such as hard red winter wheat, buckwheat or barley. Use organic soil or compost if you can, or otherwise a growbag with a seaweed base. You will also need some newspapers and plastic sheeting.

Wash the wheat and soak it for 12 hours in filtered or boiled and cooled water (the chlorine in tap water can inhibit germination). Change the water two or three times during this time.

Pour off the soak water. Place a 2.5–5 cm/1–2 in deep layer of compost in flat trays (hard plastic confectioners' trays or tea trays are ideal) and moisten it. Sprinkle the seeds quite densely and evenly on to the compost and pat down into the soil. Cut 8–10 layers of newspaper to the size of the seed tray, soak thoroughly, then use to cover the seeds. Place a sheet of plastic on top of the newspaper. Leave the tray in a well-ventilated, not over-warm room for 3 days.

At the end of this time, remove the plastic and newspaper and place the trays where they will get plenty of light – a sunny windowsill, for instance – and water once a day, making sure you do not soak the soil. In about 5–8 days the plants should be 15–20 cm/6–8 in high, standing upright and nicely green. They are now ready to cut.

Cut the grass as close to the soil as possible with scissors or a serrated bread knife. Cut grass can be stored in plastic containers in the refrigerator without spoiling for about a week; frozen it will store for longer periods but will lose some of its nutritional value.

You will need a hand or electric green leaf type juicer, not a centrifugal juicer (see the section in Juicers and Juicing Equipment, page 19). A good handful of grass will yield about 25 g/1 oz of juice, and will have a bittersweet liquorice taste. The recommended daily dose is 25–100 g/ 1–4 oz.

Rinse the trays well before starting again.

SPROUTING SEEDS IN JARS

Another way to sprout seeds is in wide-mouthed glass jars. Put the seed/grain/pulse of your choice, for example mung, chick pea (garbanzo), fenugreek, lentil or alfalfa, in a large sieve (strainer), remove any small stones, broken seeds or loose husks and rinse your sprout well. Place the seeds in a jar and cover with about 10 cm/4 in of pure water. Leave the sprouts to soak overnight.

Pour off the soak water. Rinse the seeds in a large sieve and drain them well before replacing them in the jar as too much water may cause them to rot. Repeat this rinsing process morning and night and at midday too during a hot spell.

Unless you are growing alfalfa seeds, return the sprouter to a reasonably warm place for 3–5 days, maybe under the sink, in an airing cupboard or not too far from a radiator. They grown better without light and in a temperature of about 21°C (70°F). The sprout are at their most nutritious 50–96 hours after the start of germination, but must have a dose of chlorophyll before they are used.

Alfalfa thrive on a little sunlight after two or three days: however mung beans, fenugreek and lentils are best off away from too much light. Place the sprout in the sunshine and watch them develop little green leaves, or 'tails'. Keep them moist. After a few hours in the sun most sprouts are ready to be eaten. They should be rinsed and eaten straight away or stored in an airtight container or sealed polythene bag.

ALFALFA SEEDS

Alfalfa seeds can simply be sprinkled on damp kitchen paper (paper towels) on trays and left alone in the dark. After four or five days they will have grown into a thick green carpet. Place the sprouts in sunlight for a day or so to develop lots of chlorophyll. When ready, peel them off the paper and thoroughly rinse them in a sieve (strainer). Store in an airtight container in the refrigerator until needed.

Rinse the trays well before starting again.

APPLE JUICE

Apples play an enormous part in my daily juicing routine. I have found that cooking with juiced apple greatly emphasises the flavours of other ingredients, and that apple purées (pastes) and many of our best-loved apple recipes are enhanced by the introduction of a little extra apple juice.

Apple juice added to soups, salad dressings, marinades, sauces and meat and fish dishes may sound unlikely, but the flavours of many standard dishes are greatly improved. I have found that the juice is delicious in basting roasting joints and, because of its high pectin content, it makes an ideal setting agent when making jams (conserves) and jellies, and for rescuing marmalades that refuse to set.

APPLE VARIETIES

There is no such thing as a typical apple flavour – each variety has its own distinctive sweet, mellow or tart taste. There are over 3,000 different types of apple in Britain today and over the centuries more than 7,000 varieties of apple have been recorded in horticultural journals and other literature, many in the United States during the past 250 years.

There is a distinction in Great Britain between cooking (tart) apples and eating (dessert) apples. Cooking apples are usually large, green and acidic and, because of the high content of malic acid, the English cooking apple disintegrates to a purée when cooked.

The king of the English cooking apple is the Bramley and I recommend it for juicing, or a blend of Cox's and Bramley, for all savoury dishes that require a touch of acid.

The American equivalents, Granny Smith or Gravenstein apples, are also tart and crisp, and their juice is ideal for savoury cookery. The American Rambo, Spartan or Cortland apple is fairly tart and firm and can be used in cooking savoury dishes, for baking pies, for sauces and for eating fresh and in salads. In France they have the tart Calvilles cooking apple.

English dessert apples are mostly sweet and fragrant, and sweet apple juices are usually made from the Discovery, Worcester Pearmain (the oldest English apple still in use), Laxton Fortune or Lord Lambourne. They can also enhance many cake and pudding recipes. If you have such lovely English varieties as Man of Ross, Beauty of Bath, Blenheim Orange or Crispin in your garden, you are indeed fortunate.

The Red Delicious, America's most popular apple, is a sweet mellow eating apple, and the sweet and semi-firm Golden Delicious is most versatile. So, too, is the Canadian McIntosh, which takes less cooking time, and the American Rhode Island Greening. All are excellent to eat fresh and in pies and baking.

The American Newton Pippin is slightly tart and firm, not unlike the British Cox's Orange Pippin, but it is claimed to be juicer than the European variety. It's good, too, for all round eating, juicing and cooking, as are the Winesap and Rome Beauty. The French equivalent would be the much-prized Rinette varieties.

APPLES ARE GOOD FOR US

Apples are not a major source of any one specific nutrient, but they contain modest amounts of a number of important vitamins and other nutrients. They are low in calories – a medium apple supplies approximately 80 calories. Nutritionists constantly urge us to eat more apples for the sake of our hearts, because their pectin and vitamin C helps keep our cholesterol levels stable. American studies have shown that they also protect us from the scourge of pollution by binding on to heavy metals, such as lead and mercury, and other toxic wastes in the body, carrying them out safely. Scientists contend that they aid digestion by neutralising acid, and cope with excess protein or rich fatty foods (how wise our country forebears were to serve apple purée (paste) with pork, apples with cheese, sage and apple stuffing with pork or goose, and apple with mackerel dishes).

Raw apples are prescribed for people suffering from arthritis, rheumatism and gout, and a diet of just grated apples is an effective cure for diarrhoea. An apple is also said be nature's toothbrush, cleaning the teeth and massaging the gums (however, there can be no substitute for brushing!).

APPLES FOR JUICING

I recommend the following English apples for juicing in the home juicer. The Bramley cooking apple is available all year round, and it can be used for most of my savoury recipes, perhaps blended one-to-one with the Egremont Russet, with its lovely nutty flavour. Cox's Pippin or Crispin apples make a wonderful combination. During March, April and May, when the southern hemisphere apples arrive on the market to fill the gap, I strongly recommend the New Zealand Braeburn, which also blends well with Bramley apple juice and is full of flavour and freshness.

Sweeter juices can be obtained from British Discovery, Worcester Pearmain, Tydermans Early, Royal Gala, Laxton Fortune, Chiver's Delight and John Cave apples. There are, of course, many more locally grown apples for you to savour through your home juicer, so experiment for flavour and taste.

Remember that the juice should be consumed immediately, or it will begin to oxidise and lose its potency. If you do need to store it for a little while, place an ice cube in the thermos flask and fill the flask to the very top with fresh juice in the morning so that it will be ready for your lunchtime snack or a picnic.

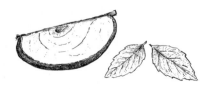

DICTIONARY OF
CONDITIONS

The following index in this chapter provides information obtained after careful research and interviews with health professionals. It is merely a guide and is not intended to replace qualified medical advice, for only a trained physician can diagnose and treat serious illness, but it can be used alongside medical advice. I have been greatly influenced in my research by Leslie and Susannah Kenton's *Raw Energy*. The authors state that 'orthodox medicine has always tended to dismiss raw juice therapy, refusing to accept that juices have useful healing powers'. Certainly some view it with a somewhat jaundiced eye, arguing that if things were proven scientifically they would by now have been incorporated in their field. However, the Kentons quote the following from a British Medical Health and Public Service laboratory publication of 1950:

> Juices are valuable in relief of hypertension, cardiovascular, kidney diseases and obesity. Good results have also been obtained with large amounts, up to one litre daily, in treatment of peptic ulceration, also in treatment of chronic diarrhoea, colitis, and toxaemia of gastrointestinal origin. The buffering capacities of the juices reveal that they are very valuable in the treatment of hyperchlorhydria (excessive production of hydrocholoric acid in the stomach).

Referring to the treatment of excessive production of hydrochloric acid in the stomach, Dr H.E. Kitchner, in his *Live Food Juices* states: 'Milk has often been used for this purpose, but spinach juice, juices of cabbage, kale and parsley were far superior to milk for this purpose.' His treatment of raw juices, both on their own and with raw foods, he claimed, cured such diverse ailments as failing eyesight, arthritis, infantile leukaemia, anorexia, and kidney failure. The climate of orthodox opinion is changing, and research continues.

The restorative powers of fresh fruit juices, packed with vitamins and purifying natural acidity, have been called 'body cleansers', and the squeezed fresh vegetable juices from sprouts, grasses and greens are the 'body restorers', brimming with blood- and bone-building materials.

The vitality and energy we instantly receive from green plants should never be underestimated for, nearly a hundred years ago, Max Bircher-Benner had a theory that green plants store the sun's energy to build up carbohydrate reserves, so that in fresh green plants we receive the very highest amount of energy possible direct from the plant, which is, of course, lost in the processing, cooking and wilting of a plant. Dr Bircher-Benner's famous Zurich clinic became a centre for diet therapy in the treatment of specific diseases and conditions, and it was here that he transformed the life of the famous American dietician Gaylord Hauser by curing him of TB. Some of the world's strongest herbivorous animals, elephants, oxen, horses and gorillas, for example, exist entirely on plant life and some Olympic athletes are strict vegetarians.

It is important to point out that most vegetables contain quite similar amounts of minerals. An essay on raw juice therapy by J.I. Rodale in *The Complete Book of Food and Nutrition* states: 'There is no one mineral or combination of minerals which is important for one organ or one disease. They are important. Even iron deficiency anaemia is not cured by giving iron, unless you give copper at the same time.'

Many people believe wholeheartedly in drinking raw juices to cure disease and maintain good daily health, and there have certainly been many success stories. However, the human body is a very complicated mechanism and it is very easy to over-simplify the process of 'cure' in one's enthusiasm for freshly made juices.

Remember that all the green juices and beetroot (red beet) juice must be taken only in small quantities and diluted with either water or carrot or apple juice as they are too potent consumed in larger amounts.

ACIDOSIS
Papaya, pineapple

ACNE
Blueberry, mango, papaya, strawberry
Asparagus, Brussels sprout, carrot, cucumber, dandelion, green (bell) pepper, lettuce, parsnip, spinach, turnip and turnip greens, watercress, wheatgrass

ANAEMIA
Apple, apricot, cherry, grape, lemon, lime, orange, prune
Alfalfa, asparagus, beansprout, beetroot (red beet), dandelion, endive, kale, lettuce, nettle, parsley, purslane, spinach, string bean, Swiss chard, tomato, turnip, watercress, wheatgrass

ANXIETY
Cantaloupe melon, grape, pineapple, strawberry
Broccoli, carrot, celery, garlic, kale, parsley, red (bell) pepper, root ginger, spinach, spring greens (collard greens), Swiss chard, wheatgrass

ARTHRITIS
Apple, cherry, prune, watermelon
Beansprout, beetroot (red beet), carrot, cucumber, fennel, kale, leek, parsley, parsnip, potato, radish, spinach, sweet (bell) pepper, turnip, wheatgrass

ASTHMA
Cranberry, lemon, orange
Asparagus, cabbage, carrot, celery, garlic, kale, kohlrabi, parsley, parsnip, radish, red Swiss chard, spinach, spring greens (collard greens), turnip, watercress, wheatgrass

BLADDER DISORDERS
Blueberry, cranberry, melon, peach, pear, plum, watermelon
Beetroot (red beet), Brussels sprout, cabbage, carrot, cucumber, dandelion, endive, marrow (squash), nettle, onion, parsley, parsnip, purslane, tomato, turnip, watercress, wheatgrass

BLEEDING GUMS
Nettle

BLOOD DISORDERS
Grape, lemon, lime, orange, papaya, pineapple

BLOOD PRESSURE PROBLEMS
Kiwi fruit, orange
Beetroot (red beet), Brussels sprout, cabbage, cucumber, spinach, sweet (bell) pepper, wheatgrass

BONE PROBLEMS
Alfalfa, broccoli, dandelion, parsnip, wheatgrass

BRONCHITIS
Cabbage, celery, fennel, garlic, Swiss chard, turnip, wheatgrass

CANCER
Apricot, citrus fruits, grape
Asparagus, beetroot (red beet), broccoli, carrot, garlic, kale, parsley, parsnip, radish, spinach, Swiss chard, turnip, watercress, wheatgrass

CANDIDIASIS *see* Thrush

CATARRH
Cherry, citrus fruits, grape, kiwi fruit, kohlrabi, radish, spring onion (scallion)

CIRCULATORY WEAKNESS
Apple, blackberry, blackcurrant, kiwi fruit, plum, raspberry
Beetroot (red beet), broccoli, cabbage, carrot, celery, cucumber, dandelion, garlic, green (bell) pepper, kale, onion, parsley, potato, spinach, turnip, watercress, wheatgrass

COLDS AND FLU
Citrus fruits, elderberry, kiwi fruit, papaya, pineapple

COLITIS
Beetroot (red beet), Brussels sprout, cabbage, spinach, wheatgrass

CONSTIPATION
Apple, apricot, cherry, elderberry, grape, lemon, lime, mango, melon, papaya, peach, pear, plum, pomegranate, prune, quince, strawberry
Brussels sprout, cabbage, celery, cucumber, dandelion, endive, leek, lettuce, potato, purslane, spinach, wheatgrass

CONVALESCENCE
Blackcurrant, raspberry

COUGHS
Citrus fruits, kiwi fruit, papaya
Horseradish, onion, spring onion (scallion)

CRAMPS
Cherry, watermelon

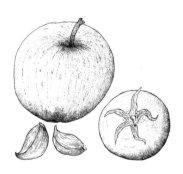

CYSTITIS
Apple, blackcurrant, cantaloupe melon, cranberry, lemon, papaya, pomegranate
Beetroot (red beet), broccoli, carrot, celery, cucumber, green (bell) pepper, kale, parsley, spinach, spring greens (collard greens), wheatgrass

DEPRESSION
Pineapple
Beetroot (red beet), broccoli, carrot, dandelion, garlic, green (bell) pepper, kale, parsley, spinach, spring greens (collard greens)

DIABETES
Papaya
Beansprout, Brussels sprout, carrot, celery, Jerusalem artichoke, kale, lettuce, parsley, parsnip, spinach, string bean, turnip, wheatgrass

DIARRHOEA
Blackberry, blueberry, cranberry
Beetroot (red beet), carrot, celery, parsley, spinach

DIGESTIVE PROBLEMS
Kiwi fruit, raspberry
Beansprout, Brussels sprout, onion, parsnip, potato, spinach, tomato, watercress

EAR DISORDERS
Grapefruit, lemon

ECZEMA
Papaya
Beetroot (red beet), carrot, cucumber, kohlrabi, nettle, potato, radish, spinach, watercress

EYE DISORDERS
Alfalfa, asparagus, beetroot (red beet), carrot, celery, dandelion, endive, kale, parsley, parsnip, spinach, sweet (bell) pepper, turnip, wheatgrass

FATIGUE
Grapefruit, kiwi fruit, orange, plum
Alfalfa, beans, beansprout, beetroot (red beet), broccoli, Brussels sprout, cabbage, cauliflower, cucumber, garlic, Jerusalem artichoke, kale, onion, parsley, potato, red Swiss chard, root ginger, spinach, spring greens (collard greens), turnip, wheatgrass

FEVER
Citrus fruits, cranberry, elderberry, grape, strawberry
Beetroot (red beet), cabbage, cucumber, garlic, onion, root ginger

FLUID RETENTION
Cranberry, elderberry, strawberry, watermelon
Beansprout, celery, cucumber, fenugreek

GALLSTONES
Cherry

GOUT
Apple, cherry, citrus fruits, grape, papaya, pineapple, strawberry
Asparagus, carrot, celery, fennel, parsley, spinach, string bean, tomato

HAEMORRHOIDS
Grape, prune
Carrot, nettle, potato, spinach, turnip, watercress

HAIR LOSS
Lime
Alfalfa, cabbage, cucumber, kale, lettuce, spinach, sweet (bell) pepper, watercress, wheatgrass

HALITOSIS
Cabbage, carrot, cucumber, spinach

HANGOVER
Citrus fruits, mango, pineapple
Carrot, cucumber, kale

HAY FEVER
Kale, parsnip, wheatgrass

HEADACHE AND MIGRAINE
Apple, cantaloupe melon
Celery, dandelion, fennel, garlic, parsley, root ginger, spring greens (collard greens)

HEART PROBLEMS
Orange, papaya
Beetroot (red beet), Brussels sprout, dandelion, endive, fenugreek, parsley, purslane, spinach, spring onion (scallion), sweet (bell) pepper, turnip, wheatgrass

IMPOTENCE
Alfalfa, kale, wheatgrass

INDIGESTION
Apple, cherry, citrus fruits, cranberry, grape, mango, papaya, peach, pineapple, strawberry

INFECTION
Lemon, lime
Brussels sprout, spinach, turnip, wheatgrass

INSOMNIA
Grapefruit, lime, pear
Celery, lettuce

JAUNDICE
Beetroot (red beet)

JOINT PROBLEMS
Broccoli, leek

KIDNEY DISORDERS
Apple, cranberry, grape, mango, melon, nettle, papaya, pineapple, strawberry, watermelon
Alfalfa, asparagus, beetroot (red beet), Brussels sprout,

cabbage, carrot, celery, cucumber, dandelion, fennel, parsley, spinach, tomato, turnip, watercress, wheatgrass

LARYNGITIS
Beetroot (red beet), carrot, cucumber, spinach

LIVER DISORDERS
Apple, citrus fruits, grape, mango, papaya, pear
Alfalfa, asparagus, beans, beetroot (red beet), carrot, celery, dandelion, endive, fennel, kale, lettuce, parsley, parsnip, spinach, tomato, turnip, watercress, wheatgrass

LUNG DISORDERS
Cranberry, orange
Kohlrabi, radish, turnip

MENOPAUSE
Blackberry, grapefruit, orange, pineapple, pomegranate, strawberry
Beetroot (red beet), carrot, parsley, spinach, Swiss chard, tomato

MENSTRUAL PROBLEMS
Cherry, grape, pineapple
Beetroot (red beet), fennel, Swiss chard, watercress

MIGRAINE *see* Headache and Migraine

MOTION SICKNESS
Strawberry
Broccoli, kale, lettuce, root ginger, spinach, sweet (bell) pepper, turnip greens

MOUTH ULCERS
Cantaloupe melon
Cabbage, carrot, celery, root ginger, spinach, spring greens (collard greens), wheatgrass

MUCOUS MEMBRANES *see* Catarrh

MUSCULAR PROBLEMS
Asparagus, beansprout, beetroot (red beet), carrot, celery, kale, lettuce, parsley, potato, red (bell) pepper, spinach, spring greens (collard greens), Swiss chard, watercress

NAUSEA
Strawberry
Broccoli, kale, lettuce, root ginger, spinach, sweet (bell) pepper, turnip greens

NERVOUS DISORDERS
Lime, raspberry
Asparagus, beetroot (red beet), Brussels sprout, carrot, celery, dandelion, fennel, lettuce, nettle, spinach, wheatgrass

PAIN
Strawberry

PNEUMONIA
Lemon, lime, pineapple, strawberry

PREMATURE AGEING
Wheatgrass

PREGNANCY AND CHILDBIRTH
Grapefruit, peach
Alfalfa, kale, parsnip

PROSTATE DISORDERS
Cherry, cranberry, pear, strawberry, watermelon
Asparagus, beetroot (red beet), carrot, cucumber, lettuce, parsley, spinach

PYORRHOEA
Citrus fruit, pineapple, strawberry
Cabbage, kale, spinach

RESPIRATORY PROBLEMS
Blackcurrant, elderberry
Leek, onion, watercress

RHEUMATISM
Apple, cherry, grape, lemon, lime, orange, strawberry
Asparagus, beans, beetroot (red beet), carrot, celery, cucumber, watercress

SCIATICA
Cherry, papaya, pineapple

SINUSITIS
Alfalfa, carrot, garlic, kohlrabi, parsnip, radish, root ginger

SKIN DISORDERS
Blackberry, citrus fruits, cranberry, grape, kiwi fruit, melon, watermelon
Asparagus, beetroot (red beet), cabbage, carrot, cucumber, dandelion, endive, fennel, fenugreek, garlic, kale, kohlrabi, parsley, parsnip, purslane, radish, spinach, spring onion (scallion), string bean, sweet (bell) pepper, Swiss chard, tomato, turnip, watercress, wheatgrass

SORE THROAT
Citrus fruit, kiwi fruit, papaya, pineapple

STRESS
Cantaloupe melon, grape, kiwi fruit, pineapple, strawberry
Broccoli, cabbage, carrot, celery, garlic, kale, parsley, red (bell) pepper, root ginger, spinach, spring greens (collard greens), Swiss chard, wheatgrass

THRUSH
Beetroot (red beet) greens, broccoli, carrot, dandelion, garlic, kale, parsley, radish, red Swiss chard, root ginger, spinach, turnip greens

THYROID DISORDERS
Strawberry
Alfalfa, kohlrabi, radish

TIREDNESS *see* Fatigue

TUMOURS
Grape, papaya

ULCERS
Mango, papaya
Cabbage, carrot, kale, parsnip, potato, spinach, wheatgrass

URINARY TRACT DISORDERS
Cranberry
Garlic, leek, parsley, watercress

VARICOSE VEINS
Grapefruit, watermelon
Asparagus, carrot, potato, spinach, turnip, watercress

WEIGHT LOSS (OBESITY)
Apple, cherry, citrus fruits, cranberry, grape, kiwi fruit, mango, papaya, pineapple, prune, strawberry, watermelon
Alfalfa, artichoke, beansprout, beetroot (red beet), carrot, celery, cucumber, dandelion, endive, fennel, fenugreek, Jerusalem artichoke, kale, kohlrabi, lettuce, parsley, parsnip, spinach, spring onion (scallion), tomato, turnip, watercress, wheatgrass

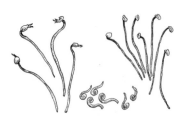

THE CANCER STORY AND YOUR DIET

No illness that can be treated by diet should be treated by any other means.
Twelfth-century Jewish physician Maimonides

It is not generally realised that there are at least 200 different cancer conditions, and that cancer can invade any tissue of the body. Some are so minor they need only to be cured by a needle prick and a few minutes' surgery, but some are so malignant they may be beyond remedy, for example the common carcinoma of the bronchus caused by cigarette smoking.

Probably the most feared of all diseases today, cancer causes extensive suffering not only to the victim but also to friends and relatives and the treatment can often be brutal. Most of us know someone who has either died from its effects or who has undergone amputation of a limb or breast, or who has suffered from the debilitating effects and total hair loss of chemotherapy treatment.

The malignant tumours of cancer occur when cells divide in an abnormal and uncontrolled manner and begin to invade the healthy surrounding tissue, destroying it by disrupting blood supply and stopping organs working correctly. Today, scientific trials suggest that people who don't take enough vitamin E and vitamin C are more likely to get heart attacks and certain kinds of cancer. Those who take enough provitamin A are less likely to get cancer, especially lung cancer.

RESEARCH

After much research around the world we now know for certain that taking large doses of antioxidant substances such as vitamins C and E and beta-carotene, the antioxidant provitamin A, and minerals such as selenium is an important weapon against free radicals, which can initiate cancer cells by damaging DNA.

Beta-carotene is the substance that makes carrots orange, and is converted by the liver into vitamin A. It is the non-toxic source of the vitamin. The American National Cancer Institute and researchers from all over the world are looking into the effect of beta-carotene on cancers of the lung, mouth, colon, skin and all other sites. Dr Richard Peto, Britain's pioneering epidemiologist, and his colleagues first suggested in 1981 that beta-carotene could be used in chemoprevention, and they must be awaiting with interest the results of the randomised Hennekens Trials, which will be of major significance in the field of chemoprevention. One trial, known as the Physicians' Health Study II and involving about 8,000 physicians, is a randomised trial of beta-carotene, vitamins E and C and multivitamins or their placebos in the prevention of cancer, cardiovascular disease and eye diseases. The study is being conducted from 1997 to 2001, with participants being followed by mailed questionnaires every six to twelve months.

Charles Hennekens MD, of the Harvard Medical School, the leading researcher on the study of antioxidant supplements, has pointed out that 'even if antioxidants could provide the benefits suggested by epidemiological studies, smoking cessation and other lifestyle factors would have a far greater effect on the rates of lung cancer and coronary heart disease'.[8] He has concluded that: 'The benefits of taking high doses of vitamin E remain to be established. There is no convincing evidence that taking supplements of vitamin C prevents any disease. No one should take beta-carotene supplements.'[9]

It has been said that we are still a long way from fully understanding the role of free radicals in the development of cancer; however, vitamin C in particular is thought to be the body's major protective element against stomach cancer. This is important because stomach cancer is one of the most dangerous and least easily detected kinds – it's often fatally advanced before being diagnosed. So it makes sense to be taking regular doses of the antioxidants vitamins C and E, preferably in the natural form of fresh fruit and vegetables.

[8] *New England Journal of Medicine,* Vol 330, pp 1080–1, 1994.
[9] Medical letter in *Drugs and Therapeutics,* Vol 40, pp 75–7, 1998.

Research studies around the world continue to show that the food we eat may be the single most important factor in the cancer process. According to researchers, 40–60 per cent of all cancers are diet-related, and are responsible for 35 per cent of all cancer deaths. The good news is that we can reduce our cancer risk, and dietary change is one simple but important step in that process. According to the World Cancer Research Fund, food additives, and even insecticide residue on fruit and vegetables, are not considered to be major cancer causes. The villains, they say, are the foods we choose to eat each day, and that is something over which we do have control.

The correct food was prescribed by the American nutritionist Jethro Kloss, author of *Back to Eden*, the classic guide to herbal medicine and natural foods which was published in 1939 and updated and expanded in 1994. For years Kloss had successfully treated cancer patients and his book cites many cases. When asked, as he was many times, what his cancer cure was, he replied: 'Correct food, herbs, water, fresh air, massage, sunshine, exercise, and rest.'

SYNTHETIC SUPPLEMENTS AND VITAMINS

Vitamin pills are not substitutes for food, and the World Cancer Research Fund and other health organisations discourage the taking of vitamin supplements, arguing that food is a complex mixture of nutrients, some of which may also be important in cancer prevention. Most vitamin pills are composed from coal tar or other petroleum derivatives; they may be chemically identical to vitamins found in fresh juices, but they have only a fraction of the biological activity of vitamins found in 'live foods' and cannot possibly be absorbed as readily as those vitamins found in natural foods.

Dr Stephen Blauer, author of *The Juicing Book*, has gone so far as to state that:

> Virtually all so called 'natural' or 'organic vitamin' and other nutritional supplements sold in Supermarkets, Chemists and Health food stores are composed of 90 per cent

unnatural ingredients, and that the remaining 10 per cent may have been derived from a natural source, such as a plant, but it certainly cannot claim to be 'organic', and it is not ALIVE.

As yet, scientists have been unable to synthesise vitamins in their labs or reproduce the live enzymes called 'Life Force'.

MISLEADING MARKETING ON ANTIOXIDANTS

A recent paper by Stephen Barrett MD titled 'Antioxidants and Other Phytochemicals' on the Internet's authoritative health website Quackwatch Home Page, cites misleading advertisements for antioxidants. He says:

> The negative publicity has not deterred manufacturers from continuing to market antioxidants as though they have been proven beneficial. Many have also responded by hyping new mixtures of beta-carotene and other carotenoids, which, they suggest, may provide the same benefits as fruit and vegetables.

And, in another quote on the benefits of using only natural foods, he says:

> Many types of pills described as 'concentrates' of fruits and/or vegetables are being marketed. However, it is not possible to condense large amounts of produce into a pill without losing fiber, nutrients, and many other phytochemicals. Although some products contain significant amounts of nutrients, these nutrients are readily obtainable at lower cost from foods.[10]

On the same subject, Ann Wigmore said:

> Many of the wild claims being made about vitamin-mineral supplements are exaggerated

---

[10] *Consumer Reports on Health*, Vol 7, pp 133–5, 1995.

and misleading. Supplements, 'youth drugs' or hormones will not, in any amount, cure the common cold, restore potency to an octogenarian, or return hair to a bald head. In most cases supplements are a waste of time and money, and they can even be dangerous in large doses ... All vitamins found in nature come 'packaged' with other nutrients to ensure their optimal absorption and use. This is the way we have been getting our vitamins for millions of years – and it is still the safest and best way to do so.

She added: 'Supplemental vitamins and minerals are a recent human invention and can create chaos in the body, especially when self administered in larger doses than those found in food themselves.'

She said that wheatgrass juice contains a full spectrum of vitamins and minerals, including the 13 essential ones, packaged with dozens of trace elements and enzymes, and is a nutritionally complete food and has never been found to be toxic in any amount whether given to animals or humans.

AN APPROPRIATE USE FOR DIETARY SUPPLEMENTS

Before leaving the subject of dietary supplements, it should not be overlooked that there are cases when dietary supplements are appropriate, especially where individuals are unable or unwilling to take in an adequate diet. For example, physicians recommend vitamins for very young babies until they are eating solid foods that contain vitamins. Other examples of appropriate use would be for those on weight-reduction diets being prescribed multivitamin-mineral supplements to RDA levels, and for children with poor eating habits, for children on strict vegetarian diets who need supplementation, particularly of vitamin B12, and pregnant women who may need supplementary iron or folic acid. Patients recovering from surgery or serious illness who have experienced disrupted normal eating habits may benefit from supplementation. Elderly people who have become sedentary or have lost interest in eating and are not getting enough nutrients can also benefit from multivitamin supplementation. To prevent thinning of their bones (osteoporosis), women should be sure that their intake of calcium is sufficient, which can be achieved by adequate intake of dairy products but some prefer to take calcium supplements, preferably under the supervision of their physician or dietician.

Dr Stephen Barrett says:

> Antioxidants have received a lot of favourable publicity. For most people, however, using antioxidant supplements does not make sense. High (above-RDA) doses of vitamins should be regarded as drugs rather than supplements. Although situations exist where above-RDA dosage can be beneficial, these should be managed with medical supervision. Most high-dose recommendations by the health-food industry and its allies are not valid.[11]

WHEATGRASS JUICE AND CANCER PREVENTION

For many years Ann Wigmore remained convinced that wheatgrass and live foods can help combat cancer. She said that – contrary to popular belief – all types of cancers can be overcome with those foods that have the ability to heal, nourish and balance the body. She did not believe that a cure for cancer would ever be found, but did believe that the body of the cancer patient must heal itself in the same way that the body recovers from a cut, bruise or common cold, and that the body must replace the lost cells with new cancer–free ones. She cited one of the guests at the Hippocrates Health Institute in Florida who had cured herself of malignant breast cancer, whose doctor had taken an interest in her case and researched many past studies of wheatgrass which had helped to make her well. He discovered abscisic acid, a plant hormone known to prevent seeds from germinating until environment conditions are right. He found from tests on

---

[11] Stephen Barrett MD, 'Dietary Supplements: Appropriate Use', 22 July 1999. Internet: Quackwatch Home Page.

laboratory animals that even small amounts of abscisic acid proved to be 'deadly against any form of cancer'.

Ann Wigmore also cited Dr Paul Robinson, co-founder of the Linus Pauling Institute of Science and Medicine, who is a keen believer in wheatgrass therapy which is still being used in treatments at the Hippocrates Health Institute. In 1983, he made a study of the various effects of live foods, wheatgrass and synthetic vitamin C on cancer in laboratory mice. The mice were subjected to exposure through ultraviolet radiation to produce skin cancer. A control group of mice received the standard balanced laboratory diet: two other groups were given the same diet and different strengths of vitamin C: another two groups received a raw foods diet that consisted of apples, pears, carrots, tomatoes, sunflower seeds, bananas, and wheatgrass. One of these groups was also given 100 g of vitamin C.

Dr Robinson summarised the findings of this research in March 1984 in an article entitled 'Living Foods and Cancer' as follows:

> The results were spectacular. Living foods (including wheatgrass) alone decreased the incidence and severity of cancer lesions by about 75 per cent. This result was better than that of any nutritional program that was tried. It was possible to duplicate this cancer suppression with ascorbic acid (vitamin C) only by giving doses so high as to be nearly lethal for the mice and far beyond any rational range of human consumption. In fact, ascorbic acid in the amounts usually recommended for colds and cancer doubled, increased by 100 per cent, the incidence and severity of the cancer.

Ann Wigmore concluded from this research that the severity of cancerous lesions in Robinson's mice was caused to vary greatly by nutritional means alone and that, therefore, future cancer research must look to diet for the answers.

In the UK, the health guru Leslie Kenton is a wheatgrass enthusiast and she has instructed people on how to grow it. Recent findings from an Israeli study by Dr Pnina Bar-Sella, in co-ordination with Tel Aviv and Haifa Hospital, actually show certain phytochemicals (naturally occurring chemicals) in wheatgrass juice that selectively kill cancer cells.[12] Surely Ann Wigmore would have been delighted at such findings.

OTHER PLANT CURES FOR CANCER

It is encouraging to learn that serious research is now investigating traditional folk medicine. A team of 15 scientists based at the Institute of Grassland and Environmental Research, near Aberystwyth in Wales, is looking at plants that may not have been investigated before and which may offer cures for the world's major diseases.

It is believed that early manuscripts containing the wisdom of ancient herbalists may point the way to a cure for cancers. In the past nettles were used as cancer treatments, for bacterial infections and rheumatism and for purifying the blood. Red clover was used to treat cancers, spasmodic coughs, burns and ulcers. Other plants were used in the treatment of TB, leprosy and common ailments such as colds and headaches.

This work has added importance now because of the emergence of new forms of disease, such as strains of tuberculosis that are becoming resistant to modern drugs. Dr Robert Nash, research director of Molecular Nature, the company looking into this research, says: 'People have not really looked properly at a large number of British plants ... Almost anything growing in your garden is likely to contain an interesting range of chemicals we know nothing about.' Interestingly, the herbal medicine pioneer of the 1930s, Jethro Kloss, also treated many cancer patients with red clover blossom and described it as 'one of God's greatest blessings to man'.

On the subject of the effect of chlorophyll in wheatgrass juice, Dr Nash says:

---

[12] Information from Brian R. Clement of the Hippocrates Health Institute.

The chlorophyll itself is unlikely to be the active component as that is of course in any plant. Fresh grass has high levels of vitamin E and so has high levels as anti-oxidant activity … However, I would expect chemicals other than enzymes to be important and no one knows the chemical composition of any plant in detail. Very minor components can have very therapeutic activity and in particular enzyme inhibitors.

Currently Dr Nash is going over old ground on the subject of 'essiac', a herbal decoction formula used by an Ojibway medicine man in 1892. It was used by a Canadian nurse in 1922 as an anti-cancer preparation, and is now available on the Internet (http://members.oal.com/essiac/indexhtn) and is widely claimed to have anti-cancer properties. Dr Nash says the four plants the formula contains are being analysed to try to understand the chemical basis for these properties. He adds that it could be that somewhere along the line of mass-production the formula has become less effective, but that variations in composition of different samples will be able to be detected.

In England, Herefordshire is playing its part in plant cures because each year my husband and I send approximately 600 kilos of yew hedge clippings from our estate to Friendship Estates in Doncaster, Yorkshire, where it is dried and then sent on to Germany to be made into the breast cancer drug tamoxifen.

OTHER CANCER THERAPIES

Before closing on the subject of cancer cures, it should be mentioned that every decade since the 1940s has presented cancer therapies that have turned out to have no real evidence of value, often causing the patients considerable expense, profound disappointment and delay in receiving recognised treatments. 'Questionable Cancer Therapy', a paper by Stephen Barrett MD and Victor Herbert MD JD, can be found on the Internet Quackwatch Home Page. The paper cites unscrupulous 'treatments' involving coffee enemas, corrosive agents, plant products, psychological approaches, mind therapies, hypnosis, drastic diet regimes, dietary supplements, raw calf's liver, the correcting of imbalances, and many more.

At the time of writing, the National Cancer Institute of America says there is no evidence that diet alone can rid the body of cancer cells. Advances in cancer studies can be made only through clinical trials, where patients are carefully monitored and the effect of a new therapy can be well documented. This may take many years of patient research. Let us hope that the work of Professor Hennekens in America, of the internationally recognised British phytochemist Dr Robert Nash, and of all the other scientists around the world genuinely working in this field of cancer prevention will soon yield positive results.

DIETARY GUIDELINES

In the meantime, we must follow the most recent report from the World Cancer Research Fund, which firmly states that fresh fruit and vegetables are now known to discourage cancer. Their dietary guidelines are:

- Cut down the amount of fat in your diet, both saturated and unsaturated, from the current average of approximately 42 per cent to 30 per cent of total calories.
- Eat more fruit, vegetables and wholegrain cereals.
- Substitute fruit and vegetable juices for some of your tea, coffee and carbonated drinks.
- Consume salt-cured, salt-pickled and smoked foods only in moderation.
- Drink alcohol in moderation, if at all.

The superstar vitamins A, C and E play an enormous part in lowering cancer risk, and they occur in good quantities in leafy green vegetables and fruit. A great deal of research has shown that vitamin A inhibits chemically induced new tissue growth on the breast, bladder and skin. Vitamin C may lower the risk of cancer in the stomach and throat. The protective powers of vitamin E, at one time dubbed by nutritionists as 'the vitamin in search of a disease', has now been found to have anti-oxidant powers. The substances found in fruit and vegetables, wholegrain cereals and pulses that are thought to help prevent cancer are beta-carotene, vitamin C, vitamin E, selenium and dietary fibre.

DIETARY FIBRE, BETA-CAROTENE AND SULFORAPHANE

Dietary fibre is now thought to play an important part in preventing constipation and more serious bowel disorders. International population studies support an association between high-fibre diets, which occur in the Third World countries, and low incidence of colorectal cancers: in Western countries, where diets are characteristically low in fibre, the risk is higher. One theory is that fibre absorbs water and increases the bulk of waste products, thereby diluting the concentrations of cancer-causing agents in the bowel, added to which the fibre speeds the movement of foods through the digestive system, reducing the time carcinogens are in contact with the bowel. Health experts recommend an average consumption of 18 g of fibre a day, and this dietary fibre should come from a variety of fruits, vegetables, wholegrain cereals and pulses (lentils, beans and peas), and should be included in a well-balanced juicing diet.

Beta-carotene is plentiful in deep red- and yellow-coloured fruits and vegetables such as carrots, sweet potatoes, tomatoes, pumpkins, peaches, apricots, oranges, cantaloupe melons and bananas, and also those that are very dark green such as spinach, spring greens (collard greens) and broccoli.

Broccoli, a vegetable from the Brassica family, which includes cauliflower, Brussels sprouts and cabbage, has highly significant amounts of sulforaphane (a compound recently isolated from green vegetables by Professor Paul Talalay and his colleagues at the Johns Hopkins University in the United States) which has definite anti-tumour properties. Broccoli is also a valuable source of iron, beta-carotene, fibre, vitamins C, E and B-complex and folic acid. So broccoli should be treated with as much reverence as the humble carrot! I like to juice broccoli with other vegetables, or blanch it for 2–3 minutes in boiling water, cool it immediately in iced water, drain it and then stir-fry it with a little grated fresh root ginger and a little finely sliced onion or garlic.

Although his theory is not proven, I agree with Norman Walker, the celebrated American nutritionist who lived to 110 years, that not all cancers are physically related. They may stem from life-long resentments or stress due to states of mind such as jealousy, fear, hate, worry and frustration. I believe, too, that such negative thoughts can lead only to self-destruction and set our bodies in a state of turmoil and on the downhill path to ill health. Many now recognise that Dr Walker, who wrote extensively on juice therapy, was a man ahead of his time.

MEGADOSING OR OVERDOSING

In recent years, to avoid overcrowded doctors' waiting rooms, people have been led to self-administration of high-content vitamin preparations claiming variously to cure the common cold, schizophrenia, cancer or hyperactivity, or to increase the ability to deal with stress and delay ageing. People have come to regard both fat-soluble and even water-soluble vitamins as safe, thinking the excess is eliminated in the urine. This is not so, according to Briony Thomas in *The Manual of Dietetic Practice*, edited by the British Dietetic Association. She says, 'ALL biologically active substances have a toxic level, and there are toxic levels in all types of vitamins'. She gives the following adverse effects: diet toxicity, induced dependency, the masking of other diseases and interaction with other drugs.

I would argue the point, too, that when taking an iron supplement it is far better simply to juice a whole orange, with its known measured quantity of vitamin C, together with its pith that helps to absorb iron, than take vitamin C in its supplement form for absorption with iron. Many people innocently exceed the recognised standard amount of vitamins, unaware of the consequences. All I am saying is that moderation and commonsense should always be exercised in the taking of food supplements, as well as in raw juice therapy. Overdosing must be carefully guarded against, especially in the use of vitamin C, excesses of which can lead to bladder problems.

THE SIDE-EFFECTS OF BETA-CAROTENE

Caroline Wheater states in her excellent *Beta-Carotene: how it can help you to better health*:

> There is only one side effect of taking beta-carotene in food supplement form ... that is called Hypercarotenodermia, a yellowing of the skin, which resembles a light tan. A yellow tinge on the palms of the hands and the soles of the feet will be noticeable if a person is consuming over 30 milligrams of beta-carotene a day.

So two to three 250 ml/8 fl oz/1 cup quantities of carrot juice daily will do you no harm. Scientists also assure us that 'there is no chance of retinal toxicity when carotene levels build up in the body'.[13] The World Health Organisation recommends that we should eat each day 'five or more helpings of fruit and vegetables, particularly green and yellow vegetables and citrus fruits', and also that at least half our daily calories should come from bread, cereals and other starchy foods such as rice and pasta.

Finally, remember that all green vegetable and beetroot (red beet) juices must be diluted in the ratio three parts apple or carrot juice or mineral water to one part green/beetroot juice. See pages 141–152 for some drink combination ideas.

CHANGE IN DIET

An abrupt change from a bad diet to a therapeutic diet with raw juices will definitely not agree with the digestion of most people initially. You will experience wind disturbance and sometimes diarrhoea, but rest assured that these reactions are the natural part of the detoxification process that the body has to make on its road back to health. In time, these problems will subside and, with perseverance, you will see signs of the responsive conditions taking effect.

Once again, may I stress the importance of drinking your prepared juices separately, never with meals – either

---

[13] Dr Leonard Mervyn, *Vitamin A.D.K.,* p 59.

half an hour before or half an hour after food – or use them as between-meal snacks.

At the end of this book are comparison charts that give you the vitamin and mineral content of some fruits and vegetables suitable for juicing. These charts are taken from the recognised standard British work on the composition of foods, issued by the Royal Society of Chemistry and the Ministry of Agriculture, Fisheries and Food. From this data you can easily work out your vitamin/mineral intake, based on 100 g/4 oz of food before juicing, and it can make very interesting reading!

To sum up, if you have cancer I would encourage you to make major changes in your diet. Perhaps 600 ml/ 1 pt/2½ cups of carrot juice a day is your best protection against cancer and help in fighting the free radicals that are attacking your body. We know that chemotherapy, radiation and surgery can weaken the immune system, and when someone is unwell and weakened by such treatments he or she needs to increase the intake of nutrients necessary to recovery. This is where a juicing programme, perhaps including wheatgrass juice, will be of value.

CANCER-PREVENTING FRUIT AND VEGETABLE COCKTAILS

The recipes for all these cancer-fighting cocktails are given in the recipe section.

Fruit Cocktails
No 5   Minted Apple and Blood Orange Juice (see page 121)
No 8   Pink Grapefruit Nightcap (see page 123)
No 21 Tropical Cancer Fighter (see page 130)

Vegetable Cocktails
No 3   The Muscle Tonic (see page 143)
No 4   Broccoli Surprise (see page 143)
No 11 The Body Cleanser (see page 147)
No 12 Carrot, Apple and Ginger Juice (see page 147)
No 13 Mr McGregor's Feast (see page 148)
No 14 Carrot and Apple Juice Lifesaver (see page 148)
No 20 The Garlic Stomach Cleanser (see page 151)
No 21 Pick-me-up Booster (see page 152)

VITAMINS AND MINERALS IN JUICES

VITAMINS

There are 13 essential vitamins that facilitate the metabolic processes of the body, for example the metabolism of carbohydrates, fats and proteins to produce energy, the building up of the body proteins, the absorption of calcium for the gut and bones, the multiplication of body cells, and the formation of blood cells. Without their presence we simply could not exist.

VITAMIN A *(Retinol)*
Fat soluble. The vision vitamin, the deficiency of which has a marked effect on the eyes that can lead to blindness or xerophthalmia. Vitamin A is found in animal foods or as carotene (which gives carrots their colour) in some vegetables and fruit. Carotene, which can be converted by the body into vitamin A, protects against cancers, in particular those on surface tissues, inside the lungs, and of the breast, intestines, stomach, bladder and skin. Vitamin A taken in excess in tablet form can be poisonous to the liver and cause damage; but carotene taken in excess can only cause a temporary orange colour to the skin, which is not harmful, so this is the safest way to take vitamin A.

Non-animal sources
Apricots, carrots, dark green vegetables such as spinach and broccoli, melon, pumpkin, tomatoes, wheatgrass

Animal sources
Butter, cheese, cod liver oil, eggs, fish oils, fortified margarines, kidney, liver, milk

VITAMIN B1 *(Thiamine)*
Water soluble. Helps maintain the nervous system.

Sources
Beans, beansprouts, cereal foods, cod's roe, duck, fruit, milk, nuts, oatmeal, peas, pork, potatoes, vegetables such as alfalfa sprouts, wheatgerm, wholemeal bread and flour, yeast and yeast extract

VITAMIN B2 *(Riboflavin)*
Water soluble. For healthy skin, eyes, hair, and growth in general.

Sources
Bananas, bread, cereals, cheese, eggs, fish, fortified breakfast cereals, green vegetables, kelp, meat, milk, mushrooms, nuts, sprouted beans and grains, wheat bran, wheatgerm, yeast, yoghurt

VITAMIN B3 *(Niacin)*
Water soluble. Like thiamine and riboflavin, niacin is involved in the process by which energy is released from food.

Sources
Much the same as riboflavin foods – beans, bran, brewer's yeast, fish, fortified breakfast cereals, kelp, kidney, liver, meat, milk, mushrooms, peanuts, peas, pine nuts, sesame seeds, sprouted beans and grains, sunflower seeds, tomatoes, vegetables, wholemeal bread and flour, yeast extract

VITAMIN B6 *(Pyridoxine)*
Water soluble. Involved in the metabolism of amino acids and necessary to help make up the haemoglobin in blood. It is claimed that extra B6 can help relieve depression caused by the contraceptive pill and premenstrual tension.

Sources
Bananas, bread, yeast extract

VITAMIN B12 *(Cobalamin)*

Water soluble. A mixture of several related compounds and needed for rapidly dividing cells such as those in the bone marrow from which blood is formed. As it is found in animal foods it is customary for vegans to obtain their supply from plant 'milks' such as soya milk or yeast extracts that have been fortified with B12.

Sources

Cheese, eggs, heart, kidney, liver, meat, milk, oysters, rabbit, sardines, seaweeds, wheatgrass

FOLATE

Needed for rapidly dividing cells such as blood cells. An increased intake is necessary during pregnancy. Folate is easily destroyed during cooking.

Sources

Avocados, bananas, beetroot (red beet), bran, broccoli, butter (lima) beans, cabbage, eggs, some fish, kidney, lettuce, liver, oranges, peanuts, raw leafy green vegetables, spinach, wholemeal bread

VITAMIN C *(Ascorbic Acid)*

Water soluble. Vitamin C has a number of useful functions. It helps keep the structure of connective tissue healthy, and it enables iron to be more easily absorbed. It also aids recovery from illness and contributes to healthy bones, teeth, gums and blood vessels and inhibits a group of cancer-causing agents. It is recommended to be increased by patients undergoing surgery, as it plays an important part in healing wounds and connective tissue (some hospitals advise patients to increase their daily dose by almost 10 times by taking 1 litre/1¾ pts/4¼ cups of orange juice a few days before the operation). An increase is also helpful for drug takers and smokers. Scientists have confirmed that overdosing is harmful and can cause excess amounts of oxalate (a calcium compound) in the urine, which can form stones in the bladder. Tablet overdosing can be harmful and the best course is to eat more fruit and vegetables, thereby getting the benefit of other vitamins and minerals. Potatoes are not a concentrated form of vitamin C, but because they are eaten in large quantities, they contribute a useful amount.

Sources
Blackcurrants, broccoli, Brussels sprouts, lightly cooked cabbage, cauliflower, green (bell) peppers, guavas, lemons, oranges, potatoes, rosehip syrup, wheatgrass

VITAMIN D *(Calciferol)*
Fat soluble. Vitamin D is made in the skin on exposure to sunlight so it can be considered a hormone. It is needed to transport calcium from the blood into the bones and back again. A level of calcium is essential for the action of muscles like the heart and to help the nerves to function properly. It is very easy to overdose in the tablet form, which can cause hypercalcaemia – too much calcium in the soft tissue – resulting in thirst, loss of appetite, nausea and vomiting and raised blood pressure.

Sources
Almonds, butter, coconut, cod liver oil, eggs, fatty fish, fish liver oils, fortified margarines, herring, liver, mackerel, pilchards, salmon, sardines, sunflower seeds, sunlight, tuna

VITAMIN E *(Tocopherol)*
Fat soluble. Vitamin E protects essential fatty acids from the destructive effects of oxygen. It is a natural anti-coagulant, aids reproduction, promotes healthy skin, and its anti-oxidant powers protect against heart disease and cancer.

Sources
Beetroot (red beet), broccoli, butter, carrots, celery, eggs, leafy green vegetables, margarine, nuts and seeds, sprouted grains, vegetable oils, wheatgerm, wheatgrass, wholegrain cereals

VITAMIN K *(Napthaquinone)*

Fat soluble. Found mainly in vegetables but also produced by bacteria in the gut. An essential vitamin for the normal clotting of the blood.

Sources

Alfalfa, carrot tops, dark green vegetables, grains, kelp, liver, soya oil, sprouted grains

MINERALS

Research into minerals as well as vitamins essential to humans is making rapid advances and scientific knowledge is constantly changing.

Mineral salts cannot be dissolved in water, so they are difficult to absorb and not easily excreted, except sodium and potassium salts and iodide and fluoride which are easily absorbed. However, our bodies do not usually suffer deficiencies, except for iron. Excessive sweating can cause cramping from loss of sodium. Most minerals in the body are formed in the bones. Minerals give bones their strength and hardness, without them they would be like rubber. The most common mineral in the bones is calcium, but phosphorous is also important and small amounts of magnesium.

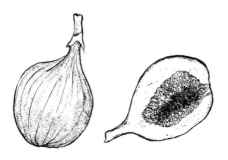

CALCIUM
Needed daily, because 70–80 per cent of the calcium in food is passed out of the body, so the recommended intakes are about three times higher than the amount actually needed. 99 per cent of the remaining calcium is transported to the skeleton by vitamin D and the remaining 1 per cent performs the vitally important function of triggering muscle contractions, including those of the heart muscles, and nerve function, for the activity of several enzymes, and for normal clotting of the blood. Crash diets and chronic gastrointestinal diseases lead to calcium loss, and high consumption of alcohol, coffee, meat, bran, salt and cola drinks make it more difficult for calcium to be absorbed. In the UK, all bread except wholemeal is fortified with extra calcium.

Sources
Bread and flour, cheese, canned fish (where the bones are eaten), dried figs, dulse, green vegetables, hard water, kelp, milk, nuts, parsley, peanuts, wheatgrass, yoghurt

CHROMIUM
Chromium is defined as a nutrient. It is part of the glucose tolerance factor, which enhances the action of insulin in carbohydrate metabolism.

Sources
Present in most foods

COBALT
Part of vitamin B12 (see page 111).

COPPER
Copper works with iron in the formation of haemoglobin and occurs in melanin pigments in skin and hair.

Sources
Liver, shellfish; also useful amounts in bread, cereals, meat and vegetables

FLUORIDE
Found in bones and teeth. Fluoride adds considerably to

the strength of tooth enamel. Adults often obtain 1 mg fluoride from tea alone each day.

Sources
Fluoride in mains water supplies, sea fish, tea

IODINE
Iodine is essential in the thyroid gland, where it is a component of the hormones produced there. Unlike other minerals, iodine is easily absorbed. It is sometimes given to those who are exposed to large doses of radiation.

Warning: do not use any iodine products available from chemists's shelves on your food.

Sources
Cereals, dulse, kelp, seafood, vegetables

IRON
Approximately half the iron in the body is found in haemoglobin in the blood, the other half in muscle tissue. Iron, therefore, is necessary for the production of red blood cells, a shortage of which results in anaemia. When anaemia is diagnosed a diet containing plenty of iron and vitamin C should be sufficient remedy. Tea hinders iron absorption, so do not drink tea until one hour after an iron-rich meal or drink.

Sources
Dried apricots, cereals, chocolate, curry powder, dulse, egg yolks, fish, kelp, lentils, liver, meat, nuts and seeds, potatoes, red wine, soy sauce, vegetables

MAGNESIUM
Magnesium is also found in the bones and is absolutely necessary for every biochemical process in our bodies, including metabolism and the synthesis of both nucleic acids and proteins.

Sources
Widespread in foods, particularly cereals and vegetables

MANGANESE
A deficiency can cause poor growth and deformities of the inner ear.

Sources
Beans, leafy green vegetables, nuts, spices, tea, wholegrain cereals

PHOSPHORUS
Phosphorus is found mainly in the bones and works with calcium, but some is needed for a chemical reaction that releases energy from food. It is more widely distributed in food than calcium. A deficiency is virtually impossible.

Sources
Baking powder, bread and cereal products, carrots, cheese spreads, dark green vegetables, dulse, kelp, meat and meat products, milk and milk products, as phosphate in dessert mixes, sausages; 10 per cent is also contained in food additives.

SELENIUM
Like vitamin E, selenium helps to prevent oxidation of essential fatty acids but, unlike vitamin E, selenium can be toxic in high concentration.

Sources
Cereal products, fish, meat

ZINC
Zinc plays an important part in wound healing. It is found mostly in the bones but elsewhere in the eyes, prostate and skin. A lack of zinc can result in hair loss and boils and swelling all over the skin.

Sources
Beans, carrots, fish, leafy green vegetables, meat and meat products, nuts, oysters, parsley, watercress, wholegrain cereals, wholemeal bread

SEA VEGETABLE SUPPLEMENTS

An excellent source of the earth's minerals is readily available to us in sea vegetables. When you consider that the ocean beds contain the most fertile soil in the world, sea vegetation is therefore one of the most valuable food supplements to be found. Seaweed roots sometimes extend 6,000–9,000 metres/20,000–30,000 ft below the surface of the water, their tentacles floating to the surface where, with the help of its enzymes and the rays of the sun, they burst forth into nodules and leaves. Therefore seaweeds, with their ability to stimulate the digestive action of the intestines, are particularly valuable as a health resource, and the carbohydrates found in seaweed do not elevate blood-sugar levels so people with blood-sugar problems can take it safely.

Seaweeds such as the large brown kelp and the edible red dulse are the most familiar. They are safe and reliable nutritional supplements that contain 12 key minerals, in particular organic iodine, which is needed by the thyroid gland to manufacture the hormone thyroxin, which aids digestion. Iodine is also needed for brain functioning, and it kills harmful bacteria in the bloodstream. Iodine deficiency contributes to enlarged adenoids, fatigue, colds and infection.

There is a wide choice of seaweeds, which are sold under the names sea lettuce, kelp or dulse, and they can be purchased in good health food stores. Fresh or dried uncooked and unprocessed sea vegetables or seaweeds are the most beneficial. After drying, they are usually crushed or ground and used in powder or granule form. By adding kelp or dulse in moderation as a food supplement we are furnishing our systems with trace elements that are necessary to our health and well-being, and which are not found in vegetables and fruits.

The powder or granules can be sprinkled on to the potassium vegetable cocktail combinations, such as the carrot, celery, parsley and spinach juices, but due to their high potency they should not be used in greater quantities than 1.5 ml/¼ tsp daily, preferably mixed with 600 ml/1 pt/2½ cups of raw vegetable juice. Kelp granules and dulse powder are slightly salty to the taste and can be added to dressings or sprinkled on salads. Dulse flakes or powder can be taken as a snack food with pieces of carrot or celery. Dulse is an important additive to meals in many countries, including Scotland and Ireland.

Other sea vegetables, which are largely used by the Japanese, are arame, hiziki, kombu, nori and wakame, and powdered kelp to make a kelp tea known as kobucha. Nori, or laver seaweed, is the type used by the Welsh for their laverbread, a green mush rather like spinach purée in appearance. It is a reddish seaweed of a distinctive shape and relatively small size, and is thought to be the most nutritionally valuable and most widespread.

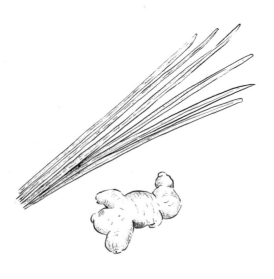

FRUIT JUICE COCKTAILS

September blow soft 'till the fruits in the loft.
Thomas Tusser

Once you have learned how to work your home juicer, the fun can begin.

You can create your own combinations of fruit and vegetable juices and bring you and your sampling friends great joy. So, experiment and devise your own drinks with what you have available, and don't forget that you can give them an individual touch by adding certain herbs, such as basil, coriander (cilantro), marjoram, mint and oregano, or freshly ground spices, such as allspice, cinnamon, ginger, nutmeg and liquorice sticks. Or perhaps you might like to add the slightly salty taste of seaweed flakes. For extra sweetness and thickening add some honey, wheatgerm, plain yoghurt or milk. For an extra energy booster, add some mashed banana or avocado.

1   Apple and Ginger Ale Fizz

The properties of apple juice are good for gall bladder and liver disorders, diarrhoea, tooth decay and loss of appetite. Apart from being a terrific source of pectin, which removes toxins from the intestines, the potassium and phosphorus in apples help flush the kidneys and control digestive upsets. This is my favourite slimline drink.

SERVES 1

---

3 eating (dessert) apples

Crushed ice

Slimline ginger ale

Cut the apples into narrow wedges, then process the fruit in the juicer. Serve over crushed ice in a tall glass, and top up with chilled slimline ginger ale to taste.

2   Apple and Ginger Pear

Pears contain a lot of pectin, a digestive aid that helps regulate the body. Pears strengthen the kidneys and they are said to be good for sleeplessness, but I would omit the ginger in a night-time drink.

SERVES 1
---

2 eating (dessert) apples

1 pear

2.5 cm/1 in piece of root ginger

Cut the apples and pear into narrow wedges. Slice the ginger root into a few pieces. Process half the apples and the pear in the juicer, then process the ginger and finally process the remaining apple.

3   Apple Juice Limeade

This will be one the most refreshing drinks you have ever tasted. Lime and lemons are a good source of vitamin C, so what could be more health giving?

SERVES 1
---

4 apples

½ lime or ¼ lemon, with skin

Crushed ice

Cut the apples into narrow wedges and slice the lime or lemon. Process the fruit in the juicer, then serve over crushed ice.

4   Apple and Orange Juice

A high vitamin C drink.

SERVES 1
---

2 apples

1 orange

Cut the apples into narrow wedges. Peel the orange, leaving on as much white pith as possible. Cut or break the orange into segments. Process the fruit in the juicer.

5   Minted Apple and Blood Orange Juice

The blood orange gives this juice a very appetising colour. Blood oranges contain five times as much beta-carotene than ordinary oranges.

SERVES 1
---

1 eating (dessert) apple

2 blood oranges

A few mint leaves

A sprig of mint

Cut the apple into narrow wedges. Peel the oranges, leaving on as much white pith as possible, then cut or break them into segments. Process the fruit in the juicer with a few mint leaves, and garnish with a sprig of mint to serve.

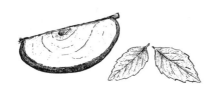

6 Hawaiian Sunrise

This wonderful drink suggests waking up on some tropical island. Pineapples contain many minerals: calcium, chlorine, traces of iodine, iron, magnesium, phosphorus, potassium and sodium. They are rich in vitamins, too, and a certain enzyme that aids digestion. Choose fresh fruit (old fruit can be woody and dry) and if you do not use all the pineapple at once, store it in a glass container in the refrigerator, but it is better to juice and consume it as soon as possible. To provide optimal nutrition, cut the pineapple into 2.5 cm/1 in thick rounds and then into strips.

SERVES 1

¼ grapefruit

1 pineapple round, 2.5 cm/1 in thick

1 eating (dessert) apple

A small slice of lime

Peel the grapefruit, leaving on as much white pith as possible. Cut or break the grapefruit into segments. Remove and discard the skin of the pineapple and cut the flesh into strips. Cut the apple into narrow wedges. Process in the juicer with the slice of lime.

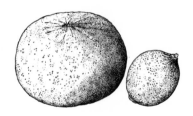

7   Kiwi Medley

The kiwi fruit, most often from New Zealand, is very high in vitamin C and rich in minerals, especially potassium.

SERVES 1

2 Golden Delicious apples

3 kiwi fruit

Crushed ice

Cut the apples into narrow wedges, and the kiwis into halves. Process the fruit in the juicer. Serve over crushed ice.

8   Pink Grapefruit Nightcap

Grapefruit are a very high source of vitamin C, calcium, phosphorous and potassium. Pink grapefruit are sweeter than yellow and contain 15 times more beta-carotene. They are good for colds, flu and sleeplessness. The most flavourful grapefruits are grown in Texas and Florida. The colour makes this an attractive drink.

SERVES 1

1 pink grapefruit

½ sweet eating (dessert) apple

Peel the grapefruit, leaving on as much white pith as possible. Cut or break the grapefruit into segments. Cut the apple into wedges and juice with the grapefruit.

9   Strawberry Fayre

Strawberries are a very good source of vitamin C and a natural sugar that cleanses the system. They are good for strengthening the blood as they are high in iron, potassium and iodine. The thick strawberry juice mixed with a little apple or pineapple juice makes a delightful, refreshing drink.

SERVES 1

---

3 Golden Delicious or other eating (dessert) apples

8 strawberries

Cut the apples into wedges, hull the strawberries and process both fruits in the juicer.

10   Aloha Delight

This drink is a tropical paradise. It is very high in vitamin C.

SERVES 1

---

1 pineapple round, 2.5 cm/1 in thick

½ sweet eating (dessert) apple

8 strawberries

If the pineapple is not organic, remove and discard the skin and cut the flesh into strips. Cut the apple into wedges. Hull the strawberries and process all the fruits in the juicer.

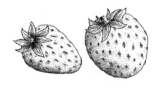

11   Peach, Apple and Grape Juice

*Grapes are said to be good for anaemia and soothe the
nervous system. Although surprisingly low in vitamin C, they
are rich in potassium and show traces of iron. Peaches are a
very good source of beta-carotene, so this combination is
extremely high in all vitamins and minerals. If the grapes are
sweet enough, the quantity of apple juice can be increased.*

SERVES 1

Grapes on the bunch

1 peach, stoned (pitted)

1 sweet eating (dessert) apple

Juice enough grapes, skins, seeds and stem to produce
60 ml/4 tbsp juice. Juice the peach with its skin. Cut the
apple into wedges and process in the juicer. Mix the juices
together and serve.

12   Raspberry and Apple Nectar

*In the nineteenth century Mrs Beeton recommended
raspberries for 'people of a nervous and bilious temperament'.
Today, it is recommended for those suffering from heart
problems, fatigue or depression, and herbalists say it has a
cooling effect in feverish conditions. This juice is very high in
vitamin C and has useful amounts of many minerals.*

SERVES 1

---

1 apple

225 g/8 oz fresh raspberries

Cut the apple into narrow wedges and process with the
raspberries in the juicer.

13   Mango Calypso

Mangoes are one of the most delicious fruits and are now stocked in most supermarkets. The largest varieties are the juiciest and they are rich in beta-carotene, potassium, vitamin C and an acid that is part of the B-complex.

SERVES 1

---

1 mango

---

1 apple

Halve the mango, remove the stone (pit) and slice the flesh from the skin. Cut the mango flesh into strips. Cut the apple into wedges and process both fruits in the juicer.

14   Morning Pick-up

A sweet and sour breakfast drink to get you moving!

SERVES 1

---

1 pineapple round, 2.5 cm/1 in thick

½ pink grapefruit

½ sweet eating (dessert) apple

If the pineapple is not organic, remove and discard the skin and cut the flesh into strips. Peel the grapefruit, leaving on as much white pith as possible. Cut the apple into narrow wedges. Process the fruits in the juicer.

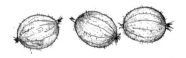

15   Apple Barley Water

A very refreshing drink in hot weather and very good for invalids. You will need two saucepans to make it.

MAKES 1.75 LITRES/3 PTS/7½ CUPS

2 lemons

25 g/1 oz/2 tbsp sugar

1 oz/25 g/2 tbsp pearl barley

1.2 litres/2 pts/5 cups freshly juiced sweet apple juice (approx 1.6 kg/3½ lb apples juiced)

Pare the lemons, halve them and place them in a saucepan with the sugar and 600 ml/1 pt/2½ cups cold water. Bring to the boil and immediately turn down the heat and leave to simmer gently. Place the pearl barley in the second saucepan, add 1.2 litres/2 pts/5 cups of cold water and bring to the boil. Strain and discard the water. Return the barley to the saucepan and repeat the boiling and straining a second time. Return the barley to the saucepan and add the contents of the first saucepan with the apple juice. Bring to the boil, then strain carefully through muslin (cheesecloth).

16   Children's Apple Juice Lollies

What could be more health-giving for children than a supply of home-made apple juice lollies from the home juicer. You can freeze them into attractive shapes and use countless other fruit juices too (if they are too concentrated and thick, dilute with a little water before freezing). Simply pour the apple juice into ice-cube trays or ice-lolly moulds and freeze.

17   Melon Medley

Melons are full of vitamins and nutrients. Cantaloupe melons are especially good for you, with beta-carotene levels reported as high as 1930 ug per l00 g/4 oz.

SERVES 1

½ cantaloupe melon

¼ watermelon

¼ honeydew melon

1.5 cm/½ in piece of root ginger (optional)

Cut up the cantaloupe and watermelon and juice with their skins and seeds and the ginger, if using. Peel the honeydew melon if the skin is too tough and juice the flesh. Mix together and serve.

18   Hangover's Harmony

Much of the misery of a hangover is caused by dehydration, so it makes sense to flush out the alcohol from your system by drinking plenty of liquids and raise your energy levels with vitamin C fruit juices. This will also replace vitamin B1, which is depleted by alcohol.

SERVES 1

¼ watermelon

¼ slice of lime

Juice the watermelon and lime and serve.

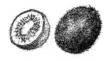

19   Aphrodite's Love Potion

Certain foods have been recommended for provoking erotic desire for centuries, particularly by the ancient Greek and Roman civilisations. Some fruits play their part in provoking desire: those that are rich in vitamins A and E and zinc are said to improve your sex life.

SERVES 1

---

1 mango

1 pineapple round, 2.5 cm/1 in thick

6 strawberries

Halve the mango and remove the stone (pit). Cut the flesh away from the skin. Cut the flesh into strips. Remove and discard the skin of the pineapple and cut the flesh into strips. Hull the strawberries. Juice all the fruits together and serve.

20   Venus Awakened

No wonder the perfumed strawberry is the symbol of Venus, Roman goddess of love!

SERVES 1

---

12 strawberries

1 nectarine

50 g/2 oz raspberries

Hull the strawberries. Halve the nectarine and remove the stone (pit). Juice all the fruit togethers and serve.

21   Tropical Cancer Fighter

Taking wheatgrass in pineapple juice with a touch of ginger is a lovely way to digest wheatgrass. A very healthy, refreshing drink.

SERVES 1

---

40 g/1½ oz wheatgrass juice

¼ pineapple

1.5 cm/½ in piece of root ginger

Juice the wheatgrass separately, then the pineapple and ginger together. Blend well together with a spoon and serve.

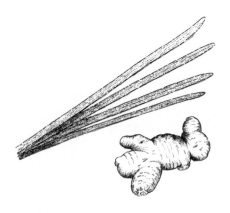

22   Apple and Cinnamon Cream

A lovely cinnamon treat.

SERVES 2

4–5 apples

2 scoops of vanilla ice cream

2.5 ml/½ tsp ground cinnamon

Cut the apples into wedges and process in the juicer to yield 350 ml/12 fl oz/1⅓ cups apple juice. Blend the ice-cream, apple juice and cinnamon in a blender and pour into two tall glasses.

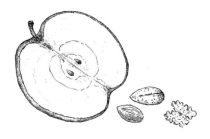

23 Apple, Banana and Yoghurt Cocktail

Remember you cannot put bananas through a juicer.

SERVES 2
2 small sweet eating (dessert) apples
1 banana, peeled and chopped
175 ml/6 fl oz/¾ cup yoghurt, chilled
175 ml/6 fl oz/¾ cup apple juice (3 apples juiced), chilled
6 mint leaves, finely chopped
20 ml/4 tsp clear honey
2 apple slices dipped in lemon juice and 2 sprigs of mint, to garnish

Peel and core the apples, then coarsely grate in a blender. Add the banana, yoghurt, apple juice and chopped mint and blend until completely smooth. Add the honey to taste and blend again. Strain the cocktail into two tall glasses and serve each garnished with an apple slice and a sprig of mint.

24   Apple and Blackcurrant Cocktail

Blackcurrants are especially rich in vitamin C, which health experts now say is vital in the prevention of cancer and heart disease. A pigment in the purple-black skins of blackcurrants is said to have antibacterial quantities, and the fruit has been used for generations as a home remedy for sore throats. You can substitute blackberries for the blackcurrants in this recipe, if you wish, and garnish with a few raspberries and raspberry leaves.

SERVES 2

---

175 g/6 oz blackcurrants

5 sweet eating (dessert) apples

6 mint leaves, chopped

20 ml/4 tsp clear honey

2 blackcurrant sprigs dipped in caster (superfine) sugar, to garnish

---

Wash and drain the blackcurrants but there is no need to string or top and tail them. Cut the apples into wedges and juice them alternatively with the blackcurrants and mint. Place the mixture in a blender, add honey to taste and blend until completely smooth. Taste again for sweetness and blend again. Strain through a sieve and pour into two tall glasses. Garnish each with a sprig of blackcurrants and serve.

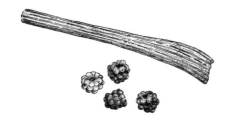

25 Iced Fruit Cup with Borage Flowers

This is a lovely fruit cup to drink poured over crushed ice on a hot summer's day. What could be nicer!

SERVES 6–8

---

1 large pineapple

7 sweet eating (dessert) apples

2 lemons

2 oranges

600 ml/1 pt/2½ cups strained weak tea

Crushed ice

A little caster (superfine) sugar, if necessary

Borage leaves and flower heads and a few slices of cucumber, to garnish

---

If the pineapple is not organic, remove and discard the skin. Cut into rounds, then into strips and dice a strip or two and reserve for garnish. Juice the strips. Cut the apples into wedges and juice. Squeeze the juice from the lemon and reserve. Cut the lemon skins into narrow wedges and juice. Peel the oranges, leaving on as much pith as possible, then juice all but a couple of segments. Mix together the pineapple, apple, lemon and orange juices and the tea. Pour over crushed iced in a large bowl, taste and sweeten if necessary. Top with the borage leaves and flowers, cucumber slices and the reserved orange segments and diced pineapple.

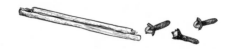

26   The London Ritz Hotel Cocktail

The head barman at London's Ritz Hotel tried several versions using Dinmore Fruit Farm's apple juices. This one was judged the best. You could use your own home juiced apple juice, from Cox's and Bramley apples.

2 parts passion fruit juice

5 parts Cox and Bramley apple juice

1 part Cointreau

2 parts quince liqueur

1 egg white

Ice

Shake all together over ice, and pour over fresh ice.

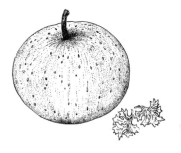

1 Apple Halloween

A healthy autumnal party drink.

SERVES 4

9 sweet eating (dessert) apples

10 ml/2 tsp light brown sugar

A pinch of salt

3 half-sticks of cinnamon

10 ml/2 tsp ground ginger

5 cloves

1 lemon, to garnish

Cut the apples into wedges and juice. Bring the apple juice to the boil with all the remaining ingredients, then turn off the heat and leave for 10 minutes. Strain. Halve the lemon lengthways, slice thinly and divide between four glasses. Pour in the spiced apple juice and serve warm.

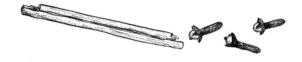

2 Egg Flip

Excellent for colds.

SERVES 6

18 sweet eating (dessert) apples

30 ml/2 tbsp sugar

2 eggs

Grated nutmeg, for dusting

Cut the apples into wedges and process through the juicer. Heat the apple juice but do not allow to boil. Beat the sugar with the eggs in a bowl until frothy and pour over 300 ml/½ pt/1¼ cups of the hot apple juice, whisking all the time. Add this to the remaining apple juice, but do not let it boil or it will curdle. Pour into long glasses and serve hot, with a dusting of freshly grated nutmeg on top.

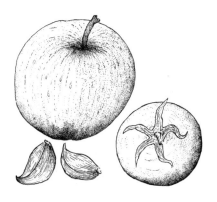

3   Hot Apple Punch

Another cold comforter.

1 orange

4 sweet eating (dessert) apples

**30 ml/2 tbsp blackcurrant concentrate or 175 g/6 oz
blackcurrants, juiced**

¼ lemon

10 ml/2 tsp clear honey

4 whole cloves

10 ml/2 tsp ground ginger

Peel the orange, leaving on as much pith as possible. Cut the apples into wedges and juice them with the blackcurrants (it is not necessary to string or top and tail them), the lemon and orange. Put in a pan with all the remaining ingredients and heat gently. Simmer for 10 minutes, then strain into tall heatproof glasses or mugs.

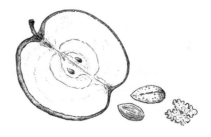

138   *7-DAY JUICING HEALTH PLAN*

4   Apple Black Jack

An invigorating drink.

SERVES 2

7 sweet eating (dessert) apples

2 cupfuls of blackberries or blackcurrants

2 whole cloves or 1.5 cm/½ in piece of root ginger, juiced

15 ml/1 tbsp clear honey

Cut the apples into wedges and juice them with the blackcurrants (it is not necessary to string or top and tail them) or blackberries. Put in a pan with all the remaining ingredients and bring gently to the boil. Simmer for 2 minutes, then pour into tall heatproof glasses or mugs and drink hot.

5   Whisky Sweet and Sour

Another cold cure.

1 part whisky

1 part apple juice

1 part sugar

1 part water

Place all the ingredients in a pan and bring gently to the boil. When the sugar has dissolved, pour into a mug or mugs and retire to bed.

6   Yuletide Mulled Wine and Apple Juice

A Christmas party drink.

SERVES 6

---

1 litre/1¾ pts/4¼ cups red wine

250 ml/8 fl oz/1 cup ginger ale

1 orange, stuck with 10 whole cloves

3 cinnamon sticks or 5 ml/1 tsp ground cinnamon

10 ml/2 tsp mixed spice

100 g/4 oz/1 cup brown sugar

300 ml/½ pt/1¼ cups apple juice (approx. 5 apples juiced)

A large wineglass of brandy, whisky or dark rum

Put all ingredients except the alcohol in a pan and heat thoroughly without boiling for about 30 minutes. Add the brandy, whisky or rum just before serving.

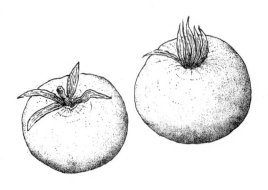

VEGETABLE JUICE COCKTAILS

My vegetable love should grow,
vaster than empires and more slow.
Andrew Marvell (1622–1678)

Vegetable drinks from your juicer are not medicines, but pure and nutritious body-building foods that feed the body with the vitamins and minerals it needs to stay healthy. Drinking them can give you shiny hair, wrinkle-free skin and firm nails. They can lower blood pressure and are said to increase your physical performance. Never drink more than 50–75 g/2–3 oz of green vegetable juice at a time. Dilute to taste with apple or carrot juice, and chew the juice, swirl it around in your mouth until it feels warm and tastes sweet which aids absorption into your system. Try and build up to two 250 ml/8 fl oz/1 cup quantities of vegetable juice a day.

1 Italian Serenade

Half a cucumber juiced instead of the apple juice also makes a good combination. It is said that there is more than 50 per cent of the RDA of vitamin C in one tomato.

SERVES 1
2 tomatoes
1 Golden Delicious apple
3 basil leaves (more, if wished), chopped
A small slice of lime
Crushed ice
Basil leaves, to garnish

Cut the tomatoes and apple into small wedges. Process in the juicer with the basil leaves and lime. Pour over crushed ice, garnish with bruised basil leaves and serve.

2   Winter's Tonic

Carrot and apple juices are the most versatile and can be mixed with all kinds of other vegetable juices. Carrot juice has a very high content of beta-carotene, but overdosing is impossible. It also contains vitamin C and B-complex and many valuable minerals. The carbohydrates in carrots gives you energy and they are good for vision, the blood, lymph and skin and digestion, so juicing carrots should be very much part of your everyday diet right from the start. The celery in this recipe is a rich source of organic sodium and therefore relieves muscle cramping. Parsley is a great blood purifier.

SERVES 1
5–6 carrots
1 celery stick
½ sweet apple
4 sprigs of parsley

Trim the carrots and cut into 5–7.5 cm/2–3 in pieces. Cut the celery into pieces. Cut the apple into narrow wedges. Process all the vegetables through the juicer with the parsley.

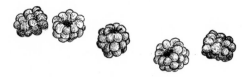

3   The Muscle Tonic

This could also be named Popeye's Favourite! Spinach is iron rich and therefore good for anaemia. It stimulates the intestine and thus helps control constipation and, like watercress, is said to be good for chronic infections.

SERVES 1

---

5 carrots

1 apple

10 spinach leaves

4 sprigs of parsley

Trim the carrots and cut into 5–7.5 cm/2–3 in pieces. Cut the apple into wedges. Process all the ingredients through the juicer and serve.

4   Broccoli Surprise

Broccoli is exceedingly high in beta-carotene, vitamins C, E and B1, is high in calcium and potassium and has traces of selenium. It also contains sulforaphane, which is said to have very definite chemopreventive powers. The American Cancer Society suggests we should be eating it several times a week, and you will reap the benefit sooner if you juice it.

SERVES 1

---

4 carrots

3–4 broccoli florets with stems

½ apple

4 sprigs of parsley

Trim the carrots and cut into 5–7.5 cm/2–3 in pieces. Slice the broccoli florets into strips, if necessary. Cut the apple into narrow wedges. Process the vegetables and apple through the juicer with the parsley.

5   Spicy Winter Warmer

*If you enjoy curried parsnip soup, you will like this drink.
Increase the curry powder for a hotter drink.*

SERVES 1
5 carrots
½ apple
¼ parsnip
4 sprigs of parsley (optional)
1.5 ml/¼ tsp mild curry powder

Trim the carrots and cut into 5–7.5 cm/2–3 in pieces. Cut
the apple into narrow wedges. Cut the parsnip into strips.
Process all the vegetables through the juicer with the
parsley sprigs, if using, and curry powder.

6   Peter Rabbit's Delight

*If Peter Rabbit had followed this recipe, he might have
avoided being caught by Mr McGregor! Cabbages have ample
amounts of beta-carotene, and they are loaded with other
vitamins and minerals. They are tissue builders and remove
toxins from the body and help digestion. I have added a little
sweet apple juice to improve the taste.*

SERVES 1
4 carrots
½ sweet eating (dessert) apple
¼ small green cabbage

Trim the carrots and cut into 5–7.5 cm/2–3 in pieces. Cut
the apple and cabbage into narrow wedges and process all
the ingredients in the juicer.

7   Weight Watcher's Wonder

As all weight watchers know, celery is a reducing aid. But it is also said to be good for nervous disorders, insomnia and muscle cramping so this is a great drink for athletes and sportsmen.

SERVES 1

---

5 celery stalks

1 sweet eating (dessert) apple

4 sprigs of parsley (optional)

Cut the celery into 5–7.5 cm/2–3 in pieces. Cut the apple into narrow wedges. Process both through the juicer with the parsley, if using.

8   Apple Aniseed

If you like the taste of liquorice you'll enjoy this drink. Fennel, from the same family as celery, is high in vitamins and minerals and is said to be good for calming the nerves and digestion. Dr Norman Walker claimed that fennel was a valuable blood builder and therefore of benefit in menstrual disorders. Its juice can be mixed with beetroot (red beet) or carrot juice.

SERVES 1

---

1 small fennel bulb (approx. 100 g/4 oz)

3 apples

Cut up the fennel and apples into narrow wedges. Process both through the juicer and serve.

9 The Body Builder

By now you will know all about the many health properties in carrots and apples, but cauliflowers are also high in vitamins A and C and many useful minerals. The apple sweetens this drink, but you could use another carrot instead of the apple.

SERVES 1

---

4 carrots

2 cauliflower florets with stems

1 sweet eating (dessert) apple

4 sprigs of parsley

Trim the carrots and cut into 5–7.5 cm/2–3 in pieces. Slice the cauliflower florets and stems into strips. Cut the apple into narrow wedges. Process all through the juicer with the parsley.

10 Fennel, Beetroot and Apple Juice

This is a colourful drink and very good for the bloodstream. Beetroot (red beet) contains many minerals, especially iron, and it is a tremendous aid to the liver and gall bladder. It's potent, so you must only juice a little and dilute it with apple juice or sparkling mineral water. The fennel aids digestion.

SERVES 1

---

1 small fennel bulb (approx. 100 g/4 oz)

¼ beetroot

3 apples

Cut the fennel, beetroot and apples into narrow wedges and process them all through the juicer.

11   The Body Cleanser

*This is the drink to cleanse the system. Cucumber juice is
very palatable and can be used to dilute green juices instead
of apple or carrot juice.*

SERVES 1
2 carrots
½ cucumber
1 apple
¼ beetroot (red beet)

Trim the carrots and cut them into 5–7.5 cm/2–3 in
pieces. Peel the cucumber if waxed, cut it into quarters
and then into strips. Cut the apple into narrow wedges
and the beetroot into wedges. Process all the vegetables
and the apple in the juicer.

12   Carrot, Apple and Ginger Juice

The touch of ginger in this drink gives it a zip.

SERVES 1
4 carrots
1 apple
2.5 cm/1 in piece of root ginger

Trim the carrots and cut them into 5–7.5 cm/2–3 in
pieces. Cut the apple into narrow wedges. Slice the ginger
root into a few pieces. Process all through the juicer.

13 Mr McGregor's Feast

After a hard day in his vegetable garden, Mr McGregor could have sat back and enjoyed a glass of the fruits of his labours! The watercress in this drink is a great source of beta-carotene and iron.

SERVES 1

---

4 carrots

4 Chinese leaves (stem lettuce)

½ apple

10 spinach leaves

4 sprigs of watercress

Trim the carrots and cut them into 5–7.5 cm/2–3 in pieces. Slice the Chinese leaves into strips. Cut the apple into wedges. Process everything through the juicer.

14 Carrot and Apple Juice Lifesaver

My favourite health-giving drink. Carrots are now said to be a leading vegetable in the fight to overcome cancer because of their high beta-carotene content. The juice combined with apple juice makes it a more palatable and a highly nutritious drink; some people drink up to 13 glasses a day. Remember an apple is a natural sweetener and is the only fruit that can be mixed with vegetable juices.

SERVES 1

---

4 carrots

1 apple

Trim the carrots and cut them into 5–7.5 cm/2–3 in pieces. Cut the apple into wedges and process both through the juicer.

15   Cucumber, Beetroot and Watercress

Dr Norman Walker, an American expert on juicing, recommended this combination for removing the uric acid of rheumatism. I have added a few sprigs of watercress for flavour.

SERVES 1

¼ beetroot (red beet), unpeeled

4 sprigs of watercress

½ cucumber

1 carrot

Juice all the vegetables together.

16   The Lung Cleanser

This is helpful in clearing the lungs. Respiratory and urinary tract infections are said to benefit from doses of watercress juice.

SERVES 1

---

1 apple

4 sprigs of watercress

¼ potato, unpeeled

3 carrots

4 sprigs of parsley

Cut the apple into wedges and juice together with all the remaining ingredients.

17   The Sex Enhancer

Several vegetables are known to be libido-enhancers, such as celery, carrots, asparagus and fennel. Celery was popular in France in the eighteenth century for its ability to increase sexual desire and improve performance. Today, scientists have found it contains pheromones, which stimulate the sex senses. Juices rich in B vitamins, vitamin E, zinc and iodine are said to give you more zest for sex.

SERVES 1
4 celery sticks
½ sweet eating (dessert) apple
¼ fennel bulb

Cut the celery into 5–7.5 cm/2–3 in pieces. Cut the apple into wedges. Cut the fennel into strips and juice all the vegetables through the juicer.

18   Hangover's Horizon

Vegetable juices high in vitamin C can quickly restore lost energy and are the answer to a hangover. Carrots cleanse the liver and kidneys and rid the body of toxins and, with the celery and orange juices here, restore the vitamin C that is so depleted by alcohol.

SERVES 1
3 carrots
1 celery stick
1 orange
A little wheatgerm (optional)

Trim the carrots and celery and cut them into 5–7.5 cm/ 2–3 in pieces. Segment the orange. Process the carrots, celery and orange through the juicer and scatter a little wheatgerm over the top, if wished.

19   The Eye Opener

Carrots, full of the vision vitamin beta-carotene, have long been renowned for improving the eyesight.

SERVES 1

4 carrots

¼ fennel bulb

4 sprigs of parsley

Trim the carrots and cut them into 5–7.5 cm/2–3 in pieces. Slice the fennel bulb. Process both through the juicer with the parsley sprigs.

20   The Garlic Stomach Cleanser

Garlic, a good source of potassium, has for many years had a reputation as a miracle cure for all kinds of ills. It has now been medically proven as an antiseptic and antifungal agent, and it helps to prevent blood clots and lowers blood cholesterol levels. It also destroys free-radicals, so it is a cancer fighter. Experts believe that one or two cloves a day are enough for protection.

SERVES 1

4 carrots

A handful of parsley

1 garlic clove

2 celery sticks or 1 slice of fennel

Trim the carrots and cut them into 5–7.5 cm/2–3 in pieces. Bunch up the parsley and push it through the juicer hopper with the garlic, carrots and celery or fennel.

21　Pick-me-up Booster

The pepper in this drink gives it a real zip, and the
wheatgrass is loaded with chlorophyll and minerals.

SERVES 1
1 red (bell) pepper
1 tomato
1 large carrot
40 g/1½ oz wheatgrass

Juice each ingredient separately, then blend together
using a spoon.

Eat an apple before to bed; make the doctor beg his bread.

Anon.

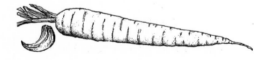

JUICE-BASED RECIPES

Here are some recipes for soups, a main course, sauces, desserts and breads and cakes using the juice and sometimes the pulp from the juicer.

Russian Beetroot Soup

Beetroot (red beet) is a powerful cleanser and builder of the blood, and this soup is soon made in the home juicer. The Russians serve it with a dollop of smetana – soured (dairy sour) cream.

SERVES 4–6

2 beetroot, peeled

1 carrot, cut into 5–7.5 cm/2–3 in pieces

1 onion, sliced

1 celery stick, cut into 5 cm/2 in pieces

1 garlic clove, sliced

1.2 litres/2 pts/5 cups beef stock

1 bay leaf

3 tomatoes, skinned and chopped

10 ml/2 tsp butter

100 g/4 oz cabbage, finely shredded

10 ml/2 tsp caster (superfine) sugar

15 ml/1 tbsp vinegar

2.5 ml/½ tsp salt

Freshly ground black pepper

A little soured (dairy sour) cream

1. Finely grate a half of one beetroot and set aside.

2. Juice the rest of the beetroot with the carrot, onion, celery and garlic.

3. Combine the juice and pulp with the stock, bay leaf and tomatoes in a pan. Add the butter and bring to the boil, then simmer for 20 minutes.

4. Add the cabbage, sugar, half the vinegar, the salt and pepper to taste and cook for a further 5 minutes.

5. Meanwhile, in a small saucepan, take a little of the stock and the remaining vinegar and add the reserved grated beetroot. Simmer for a few minutes.

6. Strain the red liquid into the soup at the end of cooking to give it a bright colour. Remove the bay leaf.

7. Serve in warm bowls and garnish each with a swirl of soured cream.

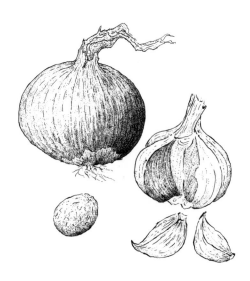

Eliza Acton's Apple Soup

Since the Middle Ages apples and meat stock soups have been part of the English repertoire, and this still continues in parts of France and Germany. Eliza Acton is considered the greatest woman cookery writer of the nineteenth century. Many of her recipes were used by Mrs Beeton in her Book of Household Management *published in 1861, two years after Eliza Acton's death. She would have been dismayed as they were never credited to her. Elizabeth David hailed her* Modern Cookery for Private Families *as the greatest cookery book in the English language.*

SERVES 6

---

900 ml/1½ pts/3¾ cups beef or mutton stock

350 g/12 oz cooking (tart) apples

300 ml/½ pt/1¼ cups Bramley apple juice or 450g/1 lb Bramley or other cooking apples, juiced

25 ml/1½ tbsp long-grain rice

2.5 ml/½ tsp ground ginger

Salt and freshly ground black pepper

Grated nutmeg, to garnish

---

1 Skim off any fat from the stock.

2 Roughly chop the apples without removing the peel or core.

3 Bring the stock and apple juice to the boil in a large pan. Add the chopped apples and cover the pan with a lid. Simmer until the apples are tender.

4 Meanwhile, boil the rice in plenty of salted water. Drain thoroughly and keep warm.

5 Pour the soup through a sieve (strainer), rubbing through as much fruit as possible, or process in a liquidiser or blender.

6 Stir in the ginger and season to taste with salt and pepper. Reheat the soup and remove any scum.

7 Spoon the soup into bowls, add a little grated nutmeg and hand round the rice separately.

Cream of Tomato and Basil Soup

The home juicer can provide many fresh-tasting soups as the cooking time is reduced. This is a lovely way to use flavourful home-grown vine tomatoes. Adjust the quantity of basil according to taste.

SERVES 4
7 tomatoes
2 onions
10 basil leaves
½ medium potato, peeled
250 ml/8 fl oz/1 cup single (light) cream
Salt and freshly ground black pepper
3 drops of Rayners 100 per cent basil essence or 5 ml/1 tsp dried basil
5 ml/1 tsp balsamic vinegar (optional)

1 Juice the tomatoes, onions and four of the basil leaves.

2 Heat the tomato and onion juice and pulp in a pan.

3 Juice the potato and add it to the pan with the cream.

4 Cook gently, stirring frequently, until the soup has thickened. Season to taste and add the basil essence or dried basil. Add the balsamic vinegar to bring up the flavours, if wished.

5 Slice the remaining basil leaves, use to garnish the soup and serve.

Bernard Clayton's Curried Pumpkin Soup

This is a delightful soup to make in October and November when you can buy just a portion of pumpkin. This recipe, described by the American food critic L.L. Waters as 'the world's best soup', comes from one of America's leading food writers, Bernard Clayton's The Complete Book of Soups and Stews. *He has kindly allowed me to reproduce his recipe here.*

SERVES 6

100 g/4 oz onions, chopped

1 garlic clove, chopped

450 g/1 lb pumpkin, peeled and chopped

50 g/2 oz/¼ cup butter

1 bay leaf

2.5 ml/½ tsp sugar

2.5 ml/½ tsp curry powder

2.5 ml/½ tsp grated nutmeg

900 ml/1½ pts/3¾ cups chicken or vegetable stock

2.5 ml/½ tsp salt

1.5 ml/¼ tsp freshly ground black pepper

600 ml/1 pt/2½ cups single (light) cream or full cream milk

30 ml/2 tbsp toasted coconut

1 Juice the onions, garlic and pumpkin. Sauté the pulp in the butter in a large pan for 5 minutes.
2 Add the bay leaf, sugar, curry powder, nutmeg, the pumpkin and onion juice and stock, cover and simmer for 20 minutes.

3 Add the salt and pepper to taste. Remove from the heat and add the cream or milk.

4 Return to the heat to warm through but do not let it boil or simmer.

5 Serve in warm soup bowls and garnish each with a sprinkling of freshly toasted coconut.

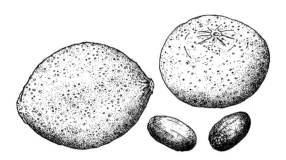

Thai Beef Curry in Apple Juice

This recipe is based on a classic Thai dish. Lemon grass is used a great deal in Thai cooking and has a marvellous lemony flavour. It can be obtained from Thai or ethnic food shops. Packets of dried stems or powdered lemon grass may be substituted for fresh: if dried it should be soaked in hot water before using; the powder can be added directly during cooking.

SERVES 4

---

60 ml/4 tbsp oil

900 g/2 lb lean beef, cut into bite-sized pieces

2 onions, quartered

2 garlic cloves, quartered

25 g/1 oz creamed coconut

45 ml/3 tbsp smooth peanut butter

2 pieces of lemon grass, chopped

5 ml/1 tsp anchovy essence (extract)

4 green chillies, seeded

300 ml/½ pt/1¼ cups medium-sweet apple juice or 225 g/8 oz medium-sweet eating (dessert) apples, juiced

5 ml/1 tsp ground coriander (cilantro)

5 ml/1 tsp cumin

5 ml/1 tsp freshly ground black pepper

5 ml/1 tsp ground turmeric

4 cardamom pods, crushed

Mixed long-grain and wild rice, to serve

1 Preheat the oven to 190°C/375°F/gas mark 5.

2 Heat the oil in a pan and fry (sauté) the beef until sealed.

3 Transfer to an ovenproof dish and reserve the oil.

4 Place the onions and garlic in a processor with the coconut, peanut butter, lemon grass, anchovy essence and chillies. Blend until smooth. Add the apple juice.

5 Fry all the spices in the reserved oil for 2 minutes, add the coconut paste from the processor and cook for five minutes. Stir into the meat.

6 Transfer to the oven and bake for 1 hour.

7 Serve with a mixture of boiled long-grain and wild rice.

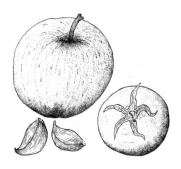

Cheese, Nut and Apple Loaf

A rich vegetarian terrine, this is good hot or cold with a wild mushroom and herb sauce, made with the soaking liquor from the porcini, and a tossed green salad. A double quantity can be prepared and some of the mixture used to stuff red or green (bell) peppers or aubergines (eggplant).

MAKES ONE 900 G/2 LB LOAF

100 g/4 oz/1 cup walnuts

50 g/2 oz/½ cup cashew nuts

15 g/½ oz/1 tbsp butter

1 small onion, finely chopped

A pinch of salt

1 garlic clove, finely chopped

25 g/1 oz mushrooms, chopped

15 g/1 oz/2 tbsp dried porcini mushrooms, soaked in hot water for 20 minutes, then chopped

15 ml/1 tbsp chopped parsley

1.5 ml/¼ tsp dried thyme

10 ml/2 tbsp chopped marjoram

A pinch of dried sage

50 g/2 oz/¼ cup brown rice

1 eating (dessert) apple, peeled, cored and chopped

1 large carrot, juiced

15 ml/1 tbsp apple juice

2 eggs, beaten

225 g/8 oz/1 cup cottage cheese

150 g/5 oz/1¼ cups Gruyère (Swiss) cheese, grated

50 g/2 oz/½ cup brown breadcrumbs

Freshly ground black pepper

1 Preheat the oven to 180°C/350°F/gas mark 4.

2 Roast the nuts in the oven for 5–7 minutes until golden, then chop them finely.

3 Heat the butter in a saucepan and fry (sauté) the onion until translucent. Season with the salt and add the garlic, mushrooms, porcini and herbs. Cook until the liquid released by the mushrooms has reduced.

4 Stir in the rice, apple, carrot juice and pulp, apple juice, eggs, cottage cheese, grated cheese and breadcrumbs and season to taste with pepper and a little more salt if needed.

5 Spoon into a lightly buttered and lined 900 g/2 lb loaf tin (pan) and press down well. Bake in a preheated oven at 190°C/375°F/gas mark 5 for 1–1¼ hours until the top looks golden and rounded.

6 Leave to cool in the tin for 10 minutes, then turn out on to a serving plate and remove the paper.

7 Serve hot or cold.

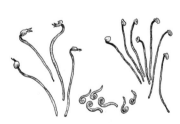

Apple Fritters for Roast Pork

This is based on a recipe from Mrs Roundell's Practical Cookery, *published in 1898. Although sweet, it makes a delicious accompaniment to roast pork.*

SERVES 4

---

225 g/8 oz cooking (tart) apples, peeled, cored and sliced into rings

300 ml/½ pt/1¼ cups water

30 ml/2 tbsp lemon juice

200 ml/7 fl oz/scant 1 cup medium-sweet apple juice

25 g/1 oz/2 tbsp butter

100 g/4 oz/1 cup plain (all-purpose) flour

1 egg white

Clarified butter, for shallow-frying

A little caster (superfine) sugar

---

1 Soak the apples in the water with half the lemon juice for 2 hours.

2 Make up the batter by warming 30 ml/2 tbsp of the apple juice with the butter just enough to melt it. Add the remaining lemon juice and the apple juice and flour and whisk to a smooth batter.

3 Whisk the egg white until stiff, then fold it into the batter.

4 Drain the apple rings carefully.

5 Dip the apple rings in the batter, then fry (sauté) in the butter until golden brown.

6 Sprinkle with sugar and serve hot.

Spiced Apple Sauce

This sauce is good with all roast meats, including duck, or with gammon steaks.

SERVES 4–6

450 g/1 lb cooking (tart) apples, peeled, cored and sliced

60 ml/4 tbsp sweet apple juice or 1 large sweet eating (dessert) apple, peeled and juiced

10 ml/2 tsp sugar

15 ml/1 tbsp Worcestershire sauce

1 Place all the ingredients in a pan, cover and cook gently for 7–8 minutes until the apples are reduced to pulp. Beat into a smooth purée.

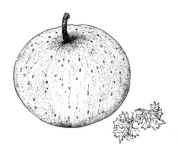

Apple and Horseradish Sauce

This recipe is from Eastern Europe, where it is served with hot boiled meats. Its sweet and sour taste is also good with a cold buffet spread.

SERVES 4–6

450 g/1 lb Bramley apples, peeled cored and quartered

15 ml/1 tbsp sugar

15 ml/1 tbsp Bramley apple juice or ¼ Bramley apple, juiced

Juice of ½ lemon

30–45 ml/2–3 tbsp finely grated fresh horseradish

A dash of white wine vinegar or balsamic vinegar

1 Cook the apples in a pan with the sugar, apple juice and lemon juice until reduced to pulp.

2 Mash to a slightly lumpy purée (paste). Allow to cool.

3 Add the horseradish and vinegar and blend together. You can add a little more sugar, if wished.

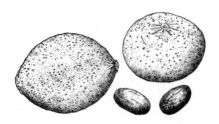

Apple Mustard Sauce

An excellent sauce with cold pork or cold turkey dishes.

MAKES 450 ML/¾ PT/2 CUPS

1 onion, finely diced

25 g/1 oz/1 tbsp butter

250 ml/8 fl oz/1 cup apple juice or 2 sweet eating (dessert) apples, juiced

225 g/8 oz apple pulp from the juicer

5 ml/1 tsp lemon juice

1 garlic clove, crushed

10 ml/2 tsp chopped fresh sage or 2.5 ml/½ tsp dried sage

2.5 ml/½ tsp chopped fresh thyme or 1.5 ml/¼ tsp dried thyme

5 ml/1 tsp sugar

25 ml/1½ tbsp Dijon mustard

1 Sauté the onion in the butter for 3 minutes.

2 Add the apple juice, apple pulp, lemon juice, garlic, sage, thyme and sugar and cook for 10 minutes.

3 Blend in the mustard and adjust the seasonings to taste.

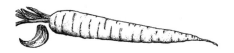

Gooseberry and Ginger Ice Cream

Many low-calorie frozen and chilled desserts can be made using a home juicer. Simply guide the pre-frozen fruits through the juicer and your cold fruit purée is ready to be consumed. We grow all the English soft fruits on the Burton Court fruit farm and I have been serving home-made ice creams in our tea room for years. With my home juicer, I can cut down on the laborious task of passing fruit through the liquidiser and sieve (strainer). I make blackcurrant and mint, loganberry, tayberry, raspberry and strawberry ice creams from freshly harvested fruit. Here's one of my favourites. The amount of ginger used can be adjusted to taste.

450 g/1 lb gooseberries

5–7.5 cm/2–3 in piece of root ginger (optional)

10 ml/2 tsp ground ginger

2 pieces of stem ginger, very finely sliced

15 ml/1 tbsp ginger syrup from the jar

100 g/4 oz/1 cup caster (superfine) sugar

300 ml/½ pt/1¼ cups double (heavy) cream

Juice of 1 lemon

1 Pass the gooseberries through the juicer (it is not necessary to top and tail them) with the root ginger, if using.

2 Blend the ground ginger, stem ginger, ginger syrup and caster sugar with the juice.

3 Stir in the cream and lemon juice.

4 Pour the mixture into an ice-cream maker and churn for approximately 20 minutes. Freeze.

Apple and Date Compôte

A delicious pudding.

SERVES 2

---

2 large cooking (tart) apples

25 g/1 oz stoned (pitted) dates, chopped

Juice and grated rind of one orange

2.5 ml/½ tsp ground cinnamon

1.5 ml/¼ tsp mixed spice

15 ml/1 tbsp runny honey

15 ml/1 tbsp sunflower or sesame seeds

---

1 Preheat the oven to 190°C/375°F/gas mark 5.

2 Peel and slice the apples. Place the slices in a shallow ovenproof dish.

3 Mix in the dates, orange rind and spices. Pour the orange juice and honey over and sprinkle the seeds on top.

4 Bake in the oven for 30 minutes.

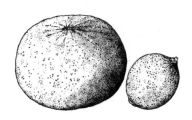

Celery, Cheese and Walnut Bread

A vegetarian recipe, and a lovely way to use celery pulp. It makes an excellent accompaniment to the cheese board for a light lunch. Celery is said to have a calming effect on the nervous system and I like the hint of caraway.

MAKES ONE 900 G/2 LB LOAF

75 g/3 oz/¾ cup walnuts, chopped

A little hot milk

100 g/4 oz/½ cup butter

100 g/4 oz/1 cup sugar

2 eggs, beaten

225 g/8 oz celery pulp

60 ml/4 tbsp celery juice

75 g/3 oz/¾ cup Cheddar cheese, grated

265 g/9½ oz/scant 2½ cups plain (all-purpose) flour

10 ml/2 tsp baking powder

2.5 ml/½ tsp salt

5 ml/1 tsp ground caraway seeds (optional)

2.5 ml/½ tsp celery salt

1 Preheat the oven to 180°C/350°F/gas mark 4.

2 Refresh the walnuts by soaking them in the hot milk for 10 minutes. Drain and chop them into small pieces.

3 Line a 900 g/2 lb loaf tin (pan) with greased greaseproof (waxed) paper.

4 Beat together the butter, sugar and eggs until fluffy. Beat in the celery pulp, celery juice and cheese.

5 Sift together the flour, baking powder, salt and caraway seeds, if using, and stir into the celery mixture. Add the chopped walnuts and celery salt.

6 Pour into the prepared tin and bake for 50–60 minutes. Allow to cool for 10 minutes, then turn out on to a wire rack and leave to cool completely.

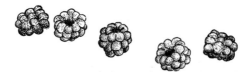

Carrot and Apple Cake

Using the carrot pulp from the home juicer gives this cake a deliciously moist texture, and the cream cheese icing (frosting) makes a lovely topping.

SERVES 12

For the cake:

350 g/12 oz/3 cups caster (superfine) sugar

4 eggs

300 ml/½ pt/1¼ cups vegetable oil

350 g/12 oz/3 cups plain (all-purpose) flour

10 ml/2 tsp baking powder

5 ml/1 tsp salt

10 ml/2 tsp ground cinnamon

100 g/4 oz finely cubed peeled apple

225 g/8 oz carrot pulp

150 ml/¼ pt/⅔ cup carrot juice or 2 carrots, juiced

225 g/8 oz/2 cups chopped nuts

For the icing:

75 g/3 oz/⅓ cup cream cheese

100 g/4 oz/½ cup butter

450 g/1 lb/2⅔ cups icing (confectioners') sugar, sifted

5 ml/1 tsp vanilla essence (extract)

A pinch of salt

50 g/2 oz/½ cup chopped nuts

2 pieces of stem ginger, grated

1 Preheat the oven to 180°C/350°F/gas mark 4. Line a 23 × 30 cm/9 × 12 in baking tray with greaseproof (waxed) paper.

2 To make the cake, beat together the sugar, eggs and oil in a bowl.

3 Mix together the flour, baking powder, salt and cinnamon and add to the egg mixture.

4 Add the diced apple, carrot pulp, carrot juice and nuts to the bowl and mix well.

5 Pour the mixture into the prepared tray and bake in the oven for 45 minutes. Remove from the oven and allow to cool.

6 To make the icing, beat together the cream cheese and butter. Add the icing sugar, vanilla essence and salt. Spread over the cooled cake and decorate with the chopped nuts and the grated ginger.

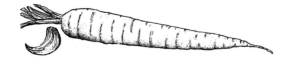

Walnut and Sweet Apple Juice Cake with Dates and Honey

I first published this recipe of my grandmother in my book The Burton Court Recipes (*Logaston Press, 1991*). *She used Herefordshire cider but the apple juice is more than acceptable.*

MAKES ONE 900 G/2 LB CAKE

For the cake:

50 g/2 oz/½ cup walnuts, chopped

A little hot milk

25 g/1 oz/1 tbsp butter

100 g/4 oz/1 cup sugar

2 eggs, thoroughly beaten

5 ml/1 tsp bicarbonate of soda (baking soda)

5 ml/1 tsp grated nutmeg

225 g/8 oz/2 cups plain (all-purpose) flour

250 ml/8 fl oz/1 cup sweet apple juice or 3 sweet eating (dessert) apples, juiced

For the filling and topping:

100 g/4 oz/½ cup butter

10 ml/2 tsp soya flour or grated nuts

75 g/3 oz dates, chopped

30 ml/2 tbsp clear honey

A squeeze of lemon juice

Sifted icing (confectioners') sugar, for glazing

A few walnut halves and halved glacé (candied) cherries, to decorate

1 Preheat the oven to 180°C/350°F/gas mark 4. Grease a 900 g/2 lb loaf tin (pan) and line with greaseproof (waxed) paper.

2 To make the cake, refresh the walnuts by placing them in the hot milk and leaving to stand for 10 minutes. Drain.

3 Cream together the butter and sugar and add the eggs and walnuts.

4 Sift together the baking soda, nutmeg and half the plain flour and add to the egg mixture.

5 Pour over the apple juice, beat to a froth and mix thoroughly.

6 Stir in the remaining flour, turn into the prepared tin and bake in the oven for 45 minutes.

7 Remove the cake from the oven, turn out on to a wire rack and leave to cool.

8 To make the filling, cream the butter thoroughly, add the soya flour or grated nuts, the dates, honey and lemon juice.

9 When cold, split the cake into three horizontally and sandwich together with the filling. Mix the icing sugar with a little water and spread over the cake to glaze. Decorate the top with walnuts halves and halved glacé cherries.

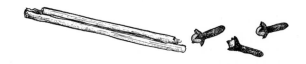

Orange and Date Wholemeal Loaf

A healthy buttered loaf.

MAKES ONE 900 G/2 LB LOAF

225 g/8 oz pitted (stoned) dates, chopped

100/4 oz/1 cup caster (superfine) sugar

A pinch of salt

5 ml/1 tsp bicarbonate of soda (baking soda)

Grated rind of 2 oranges

50 g/2 oz/¼ cup margarine

175 ml/6 fl oz/¾ cup orange juice (approx. 2 oranges, juiced)

1 egg, beaten

225 g/8 oz/2 cups self-raising (self-rising) wholemeal flour

5 ml/1 tsp vanilla essence (extract)

1 Preheat the oven to 160°C/325°F/gas mark 3. Grease a 900 g/2 lb loaf tin (pan) and base line with greaseproof (waxed) paper.

2 Place the dates, sugar, salt, bicarbonate of soda and orange rind in a mixing bowl.

3 Melt the margarine in a small saucepan. Add the orange juice and pour over the dry ingredients. Mix well and allow to cool a little.

4 Add the egg, flour and vanilla essence and mix to a smooth batter.

5 Pour the mixture into the prepared tin and bake in the centre of the oven for approximately 1¼ hours until firm.

6 Turn out on to a wire rack and leave to cool. Eat cold, sliced and buttered.

COMPARISON CHARTS OF THE NUTRITIONAL CONTENT OF FRUITS AND VEGETABLES

The following data has been taken from *The Composition of Foods*, by courtesy of the Royal Society of Chemistry and the Ministry of Agriculture, Fisheries and Food. The charts show the composition of whole raw fruits and vegetables weighing 100 g/4 oz before being juiced.

Don't be daunted by such lists of figures. For the most interesting reading, follow the line indicated for each item, for instance, on the vitamin pages find the amount of beta-carotene (vitamin A) that is given for carrots, spinach, the outer leaves of cabbages and lettuces, and compare the figures with that for pink and white grapefruit and apricots, blood oranges, cantaloupe melons, mangoes and turnip tops (all cancer-fighting fruits and vegetables). Also, on the mineral pages, note the amount of minerals that can be found in 100 g/4 oz of parsley and watercress, and the potassium in prunes!

N indicates that a nutrient is present in significant quantities but there is no reliable information on the amount.

Tr indicates trace.

Figures in brackets indicate an estimated value.

Data relates to quantities per 100 g/4 oz of whole raw fruits or vegetables before being juiced.

Food	Carotene µg	Vitamin D µg	Vitamin E mg	Thiamin mg	Riboflavin mg	Niacin mg	Tryptophan mg	Vitamin B6 mg	Vitamin B12 µg	Folate µg	Pantothenate mg	Biotin µg	Vitamin C mg
Alfalfa sprouts	(96)	0	N	0.04	0.06	0.5	0.6	0.03	0	36	0.56	N	2
Apples, cooking, peeled (Unpeeled cooking apples contain 20 mg vitamin C per 100 g/4 oz.)	(17)	0	0.27	0.04	0.02	0.1	0.1	0.06	0	5	Tr	1.2	14
Apples, eating, average	18	0	0.59	0.03	0.02	0.1	0.1	0.06	0	1	Tr	1.2	6
Apples, Cox's Pippin	(18)	0	0.59	0.03	0.03	0.2	0.1	0.08	0	4	Tr	1.2	9
Apples, Golden Delicious	15	0	0.59	0.03	0.03	0.1	0.1	0.11	0	1	Tr	1.2	4
Apples, Granny Smith	5	0	0.59	0.04	0.02	0.1	0.1	0.08	0	1	Tr	1.2	4
Apples, red dessert (Storage may considerably affect vitamin C levels in all apples.)	15	0	0.59	0.03	0.02	0.1	0.1	0.04	0	1	Tr	1.2	3
Apricots	405	0	N	0.04	0.05	0.5	0.1	0.08	0	5	0.24	N	6
Artichoke, Jerusalem (boiled in unsalted water)													
Asparagus	315	0	1.16	0.16	0.06	1.0	0.5	0.09	0	175	0.17	(0.4)	12
Beansprouts, mung	40	0	N	0.11	0.04	0.5	0.5	0.10	0	61	0.38	N	7
Beans, green or French	(330)	0	0.20	0.05	0.07	0.9	0.5	0.05	0	(80)	0.09	1.0	12
Beetroot (beet)	20	0	Tr	0.01	0.01	0.1	0.3	0.03	0	150	0.12	Tr	5
Blackberries	80	0	2.37	0.02	0.05	0.5	0.1	0.05	0	34	0.25	0.4	15
Blackcurrants (Levels of vitamin C in blackcurrants ranged from 150 to 230 mg per 100 g/4 oz.)	100	0	1.00	0.03	0.06	0.3	0.1	0.08	0	N	0.40	2.4	200
Broccoli, green	575	0	(1.30)	0.10	0.06	0.9	0.8	0.14	0	90	N	N	87
Brussels sprouts	215	0	1.00	0.15	0.11	0.2	0.7	0.37	0	135	1.00	0.4	115
Cabbage, average	385	0	0.20	0.15	0.02	0.5	0.3	0.17	0	75	0.21	0.1	49
Cabbage, Chinese	70	0	N	0.09	Tr	0.2	0.2	0.11	0	77	0.11	Tr	21
Cabbage, January King	340	0	0.20	0.22	0.02	0.3	0.3	0.22	0	78	0.21	0.1	49
Cabbage, red	15	0	0.20	0.02	0.01	0.4	0.2	0.09	0	39	0.32	0.1	55
Cabbage, Savoy	995	0	0.20	0.15	0.03	0.7	0.3	0.19	0	150	0.21	0.1	62
Cabbage, summer	200	0	0.20	0.11	0.03	0.7	0.3	0.09	0	40	0.21	0.1	48
Cabbage, white (The amount of carotene in leafy vegetables depends on the amount of chlorophyll, and the outer green leaves may contain 50 times as much as inner white ones. This is the value for inner leaves. Outer leaves contain α-tocopherol per 100 g/4 oz)	40	0	0.20	0.12	0.01	0.3	0.2	0.18	0	34	0.21	0.1	35
Carrots, old	8115	0	0.56	0.10	0.01	0.2	0.1	0.14	0	12	0.25	0.6	6
Carrots, young (Levels of carotene in carrots ranged from 4300 to 11000 µg per 100 g/4 oz.)	5330	0	(0.56)	0.04	0.02	0.2	0.1	0.07	0	28	(0.25)	(0.6)	4
Celery	50	0	0.20	0.06	0.01	0.3	0.1	0.03	0	16	0.40	0.1	8
Cherries	25	0	0.13	0.03	0.03	0.2	0.1	0.05	0	5	0.26	0.4	11

Food	Carotene µg	Vitamin D µg	Vitamin E mg	Thiamin mg	Riboflavin mg	Niacin mg	Tryptophan mg	Vitamin B6 mg	Vitamin B12 µg	Folate µg	Pantothenate mg	Biotin µg	Vitamin C mg
Cucumber	60	0	0.07	0.03	0.01	0.2	0.1	0.04	0	9	0.30	0.9	2
(Levels of carotene in cucumber can be as high as 260 µg per 100 g/4 oz. In peeled cucumbers, the carotine ranges from 0 to 35 µg per 100 g/4 oz.)													
Cranberries	22	0	N	0.03	0.02	0.1	0.1	0.07	0	2	0.22	N	13
Elderberries	(360)	0	N	0.07	0.07	1.0	0.1	0.24	0	17	0.16	1.8	27
Fennel, Florence	140	0	N	0.06	0.01	0.6	N	0.06	0	42	N	N	5
Garlic	Tr	0	0.01	0.13	0.03	0.3	1.9	0.38	0	5	N	N	17
Grapes	17	0	Tr	0.05	0.01	0.2	Tr	0.10	0	2	0.05	0.3	3
Grapefruit	17	0	(0.19)	0.05	0.02	0.3	0.1	0.03	0	26	0.28	(1.0)	36
(Pink varieties of grapefruit contain approximately 280 µg of carotene per 100 g/4 oz.)													
Kale, curly	3145	0	(1.70)	0.08	0.09	1.0	0.7	0.26	0	120	0.09	0.5	110
Kiwi fruit	37	0	N	0.01	0.03	0.3	0.3	0.15	0	N	N	N	59
Kohlrabi	Tr	0	Tr	0.11	Tr	0.3	0.2	0.10	0	82	0.17	N	43
Leeks	735	0	0.92	0.29	0.05	0.4	0.2	0.48	0	56	0.12	1.4	17
Lemons, whole without pips	18	0	N	0.05	0.04	0.2	0.1	0.11	0	N	0.23	0.5	58
Lettuce, average	355	0	0.57	0.12	0.02	0.4	0.1	0.04	0	55	(0.18)	0.17	5
Lettuce, butterhead	910	0	0.57	0.15	0.03	0.5	0.1	0.08	0	57	0.18	0.7	7
Lettuce, cos	290	0	0.57	0.12	0.02	0.6	0.1	0.03	0	55	(0.18)	0.7	5
Lettuce, iceberg	50	0	0.57	0.11	0.01	0.3	0.1	0.03	0	53	(0.18)	0.7	3
Lettuce, Webbs	180	0	0.57	0.11	0.01	0.3	0.1	0.03	0	56	(0.18)	0.7	5
(Carotene in lettuce are average figures. The outer green leaves may contain 50 times as much carotene as the inner white ones.)													
Limes, peeled	12	0	N	0.03	0.02	0.2	0.1	(0.08)	0	8	0.22	N	46
Mangoes, ripe	1800	0	1.05	0.04	0.05	0.5	1.3	0.13	0	N	0.16	N	37
(Levels of carotene in mangoes ranged from 300 to 3000 µg per 100 g/4 oz.)													
Melon, average	N	0	0.10	0.03	0.01	0.4	Tr	0.09	0	3	0.17	N	17
Melon, canteloupe	1000	0	0.10	0.04	0.02	0.6	Tr	0.11	0	5	0.13	N	26
Melon, galia	N	0	(0.10)	(0.03)	(0.01)	(0.4)	Tr	(0.09)	0	(3)	(0.17)	N	15
Melon, honeydew	48	0	0.10	0.03	0.01	0.3	Tr	0.06	0	2	0.21	N	9
Melon, watermelon	230	0	(0.10)	0.05	0.01	0.1	Tr	0.14	0	2	0.21	1.0	8
(The carotene level is an average value. Carotene levels have been reported for rock melons at 835 µg and for canteloupe melons at 1510 to 1930 µg per 100 g/4 oz)													
Onions	10	0	0.31	0.13	Tr	0.7	0.3	0.20	0	17	0.11	0.9	5
Oranges	28	0	0.24	0.11	0.04	0.4	0.1	0.10	0	31	0.37	1.0	54
(Blood oranges have been found to contain 155 µg carotene per 100 g/4 oz.)													
Papaya (paw paw)	810	0	N	0.03	0.04	0.3	0.1	0.03	0	1	0.22	N	60
Parsley	4040	0	1.70	0.23	0.06	1.0	0.5	0.09	0	170	0.30	0.4	190
Parsnip	30	0	1.00	0.23	0.01	1.0	0.5	0.11	0	87	0.50	0.1	17
Peaches	58	0	N	0.02	0.04	0.6	0.2	0.02	0	3	0.17	(0.2)	31

Food	Carotene µg	Vitamin D µg	Vitamin E mg	Thiamin mg	Riboflavin mg	Niacin mg	Tryptophan mg	Vitamin B6 mg	Vitamin B12 µg	Folate µg	Pantothenate mg	Biotin µg	Vitamin C mg
Pears, average	18	0	0.50	0.02	0.03	0.2	Tr	0.02	0	2	0.07	0.2	6
Pears, Comice	15	0	0.50	0.02	0.03	0.2	Tr	0.2	0	2	0.07	0.2	6
Pears, Conference	15	0	0.50	0.02	0.03	0.2	Tr	0.2	0	2	0.07	0.2	6
Pears, William	25	0	0.50	0.02	0.03	0.2	Tr	0.02	0	2	0.07	0.2	6
Pineapple	18	0	0.10	0.08	0.03	0.3	0.1	0.09	0	5	0.16	0.3	12
Plums, average	295	0	0.61	0.05	0.03	1.1	0.1	0.05	0	3	0.15	Tr	4
Prunes	155	0	N	0.10	0.20	1.5	0.5	0.24	0	4	0.46	Tr	Tr
Potatoes, early new	Tr	0	(0.06)	0.15	0.02	0.4	0.4	(0.44)	0	25	(0.37)	(0.3)	16
Potatoes, main crop, average (Freshly dug potatoes contain 21 mg of vitamin C per 100 g/ 4 oz. This falls to 9 mg per 100 g/4 oz after three months' storage and to 7 mg after nine months.)	Tr	0	0.06	0.21	0.02	0.6	0.5	0.44	0	35	0.37	0.3	11
Radishes	Tr	0	0	0.03	Tr	0.4	0.1	0.07	0	38	0.18	N	17
Raspberries	6	0	0.48	0.03	0.05	0.5	0.3	0.06	0	33	0.24	1.9	32
Spinach	3535	0	1.71	0.07	0.09	1.2	0.7	0.17	0	150	(0.27)	(0.1)	26
Spring onions (scallions) (bulbs and tops)	620	0	N	0.05	0.03	0.5	0.5	0.13	0	54	0.07	N	26
Strawberries	8	0	0.20	0.03	0.03	0.6	0.1	0.06	0	20	0.34	11	77
Tomatoes	640	0	1.22	0.09	0.01	1.0	0.1	0.14	0	17	0.25	1.5	17
Turnip	20	0	Tr	0.05	0.01	0.4	0.2	0.08	0	14	0.20	0.1	17
Turnip tops (boiled in unsalted water)	(6000)	0	2.87	0.06	0.20	0.5	0.6	0.18	0	120	0.27	(0.4)	40
Watercress	2520	0	1.46	0.16	0.06	0.3	0.5	0.23	0	N	0.10	0.4	62

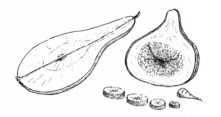

Data relates to quantities per 100 g/4 oz of whole raw fruits or vegetables before being juiced.

Food	Sodium mg	Potassium mg	Calcium mg	Magnesium mg	Phosphorus mg	Iron mg	Copper mg	Zinc mg	Sulphur mg	Chloride mg	Manganese mg	Selenium µg	Iodine µg
Alfalfa sprouts	6	79	32	27	70	1.0	0.16	0.9	N	N	0.2	N	N
Apples, cooking, peeled	2	88	4	3	7	0.1	0.02	Tr	3	2	Tr	Tr	Tr
Apples, eating, average	3	120	4	5	11	0.1	0.02	0.1	6	Tr	0.1	Tr	Tr
Apples, Cox's Pippin	3	130	4	6	12	0.2	Tr	Tr	6	Tr	Tr	Tr	Tr
Apples, Golden Delicious	4	110	4	5	9	0.2	0.04	0.1	6	Tr	0.1	Tr	Tr
Apples, Granny Smith	2	120	4	4	9	0.1	0.02	Tr	6	1	0.1	Tr	Tr
Apples, red dessert	1	110	4	5	10	0.1	0.04	Tr	6	Tr	Tr	Tr	Tr
Apricots	2	270	15	11	20	0.5	0.06	0.1	6	3	0.1	(1)	N
Artichoke, Jerusalem (boiled in unsalted water)	3	420	30	11	33	0.4	0.12	0.1	22	58	N	N	N
Asparagus	1	260	27	13	72	0.7	0.08	0.7	47	60	0.2	(1)	Tr
Beansprouts, mung	5	74	20	18	48	1.7	0.08	0.3	N	15	0.3	N	N
Beans, green or French	Tr	230	36	17	38	1.2	0.01	0.2	17	9	N	N	N
Beetroot (beet)	66	380	20	11	51	1.0	0.02	0.4	16	59	0.7	Tr	N
Blackberries	2	160	41	23	31	0.7	0.11	0.2	9	22	1.4	Tr	N
Blackcurrants	3	370	60	17	43	1.3	0.14	0.3	33	15	0.3	N	N
Broccoli, green	8	370	56	22	87	1.7	0.02	0.6	130	100	0.2	Tr	2
Brussels sprouts	6	450	26	8	77	0.7	0.02	0.5	93	38	0.2	N	1
Cabbage, average	5	270	52	8	41	0.7	0.02	0.3	N	37	0.2	(1)	2
Cabbage, Chinese	7	230	54	7	27	0.6	0.02	0.2	N	18	0.3	N	N
Cabbage, January King	3	270	68	6	46	0.6	0.02	0.4	N	45	0.2	(2)	2
Cabbage, red	8	250	60	9	37	0.4	0.01	0.1	68	45	0.2	(2)	(2)
Cabbage, Savoy	5	320	53	7	44	1.1	0.03	0.3	88	48	0.2	(2)	2
Cabbage, summer	7	240	38	12	35	0.4	0.01	0.1	N	14	0.2	(2)	2
Cabbage, white	7	240	49	6	29	0.5	0.01	0.2	54	40	0.2	Tr	2
Carrots, old	25	170	25	3	15	0.3	0.02	0.1	7	33	0.1	1	2
Carrots, young	40	240	34	9	25	0.4	0.02	0.2	(7)	39	(0.1)	(1)	(2)
Celery	60	320	41	5	21	0.4	0.01	0.1	15	130	0.1	(3)	N
Cherries	1	210	13	10	21	0.2	0.07	0.1	7	Tr	0.1	(1)	Tr
Cucumber	3	140	18	8	49	0.3	0.01	0.1	11	17	0.1	Tr	3
Cranberries	2	95	12	7	11	0.7	0.05	0.2	11	Tr	0.1	Tr	N
Elderberries	1	290	37	0	48	1.6	N	N	N	N	N	N	N
Fennel, Florence	11	440	24	8	26	0.3	0.02	0.5	N	27	N	N	N
Garlic	4	620	19	25	170	1.9	0.06	1.0	N	73	0.5	2	3
Grapes, average	2	210	13	7	18	0.3	0.12	0.1	8	Tr	0.1	(1)	1
Grapefruit	3	200	23	9	20	0.1	0.02	Tr	7	3	Tr	(1)	N
Kale, curly	43	450	130	34	61	1.7	0.03	0.4	N	68	.8	(2)	N
Kiwi Fruit	4	290	25	15	32	0.4	0.13	0.1	16	39	0.1	N	N
Kohlrabi	4	340	30	10	35	0.3	Tr	0.1	N	34	0.1	N	1
Leeks	2	260	24	3	44	1.1	0.02	0.2	58	59	0.2	(1)	N
Lemons, whole without pips	5	150	85	12	18	0.5	0.26	0.1	12	5	N	(1)	N
Lettuce, average	3	220	28	6	28	0.7	0.01	0.2	16	47	0.3	(1)	2
Lettuce, butterhead	5	360	53	8	43	1.5	0.04	0.4	16	67	0.3	(1)	2
Lettuce, cos	1	220	21	6	29	0.6	Tr	0.2	16	48	0.3	(1)	2
Lettuce, iceberg	2	160	19	5	18	0.4	0.01	0.1	16	42	0.3	(1)	2
Lettuce, Webbs	4	150	20	5	21	0.5	0.01	0.1	16	29	0.3	(1)	2
Limes, peeled	2	130	23	11	18	0.4	0.05	0.1	N	N	Tr	N	N

Food	Sodium mg	Potassium mg	Calcium mg	Magnesium mg	Phosphorus mg	Iron mg	Copper mg	Zinc mg	Sulphur mg	Chloride mg	Manganese mg	Selenium μg	Iodine μg
Mangoes, ripe	2	180	12	13	16	0.7	0.12	0.1	N	N	0.3	N	N
Melon, average	24	190	14	11	13	0.2	Tr	Tr	9	55	Tr	Tr	N
Melon, canteloupe	8	210	20	11	13	0.3	Tr	Tr	12	44	Tr	Tr	(4)
Melon, galia	31	150	13	12	10	0.2	Tr	0.1	9	75	Tr	Tr	N
Melon, honeydew	32	210	9	10	16	0.1	Tr	Tr	6	45	Tr	Tr	N
Melon, watermelon	2	100	7	8	9	0.3	0.03	0.2	N	N	Tr	Tr	Tr
Onions	3	160	25	4	30	0.3	0.05	0.2	51	25	0.1	(1)	3
Oranges	5	150	47	10	21	0.1	0.05	0.1	10	3	Tr	(1)	2
Papaya (paw paw)	5	200	23	11	13	0.5	0.08	0.2	13	11	0.1	N	N
Parsley	33	760	200	23	64	7.7	0.03	0.7	N	160	0.2	(1)	N
Parsnip	10	450	41	23	74	0.6	0.05	0.3	17	49	0.5	2	N
Peaches	1	160	7	9	22	0.4	0.06	0.1	6	Tr	0.1	(1)	3
Pears, average	3	150	11	7	13	0.2	0.06	0.1	5	1	Tr	Tr	1
Pears, Comice	3	150	12	7	13	0.2	0.04	0.1	5	Tr	Tr	Tr	1
Pears, Conference	4	150	11	7	13	0.2	0.06	0.1	5	2	Tr	Tr	1
Pears, William	2	150	9	8	12	0.1	0.08	0.2	5	1	0.1	Tr	1
Pineapple	2	160	18	16	10	0.2	0.11	0.1	3	29	0.5	Tr	Tr
Plums, average	2	240	13	8	23	0.4	0.10	0.1	5	Tr	0.1	Tr	Tr
Prunes	12	860	38	27	83	2.9	0.16	0.5	19	3	0.3	3	N
Potatoes, early new	11	320	6	14	34	0.3	0.09	0.20	(30)	57	(0.1)	(1)	(3)
Potatoes, main crop	7	360	5	17	37	0.4	0.08	0.3	30	66	0.1	1	3
Radishes, red	11	240	19	5	20	0.6	0.01	0.2	38	37	0.1	(2)	(1)
Raspberries	3	170	25	19	31	0.7	0.10	0.3	17	22	0.4	N	N
Spinach	140	500	170	54	45	2.1	0.04	0.7	20	98	0.6	(1)	2
Spring onions (scallions) (bulbs and tops)	7	260	39	12	29	1.9	0.06	0.4	(50)	31	0.2	N	N
Strawberries	6	160	16	10	24	0.4	0.07	0.1	13	18	0.3	Tr	9
Tomatoes	9	250	7	7	24	0.5	0.01	0.1	11	55	0.1	Tr	2
Turnip	15	280	48	8	41	0.2	0.01	0.1	22	39	0.1	(1)	N
Turnips tops (boiled in unsalted water)	7	78	98	10	45	3.1	0.09	0.4	39	15	N	N	N
Watercress	49	230	170	15	52	2.2	0.01	0.7	100	170	0.6	N	N

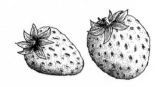

USEFUL ADDRESSES

Organic Directory Magazine
Green Books
Foxhole
Dartington
Totnes
Devon TQ9 6EB
Tel: 01803 863260

Planet Organic Ltd
42 Westbourne Grove
London W2 5SH
Tel: 0207 221 7171; fax 0171 221 1923

Malcolm Simmonds Herbal Supplies
3 Burton Villas
Hove
East Sussex BN3 6FN
Tel: 01273 202401
(suppliers of wheatgrass juice in powder form)

Organic Foods Magazine, published by The Soil
Association
The Organic Food and Farming Centre
86 Colston Street
Bristol BS1 5BB
(updated National Directory of farm shops and box schemes)

The Nutri Centre
7 Park Crescent
London W1N 3HE
Tel: 0207 436 5122
(ground floor of the Hale clinic – suppliers of healthcare
products)

Organics Direct
1–7 Willow Street
London EC2A 4BH
Tel: 0207 729 2828

Biocare
54 Northfield Road
Kings Norton
Birmingham
B30 1JH
Tel: 0121 433 3727
(nutritional healthcare products)

The Society of Complementary Medicine
31 Weymouth Street
London W1N 3FJ
Tel: 0207 436 0821

Christopher McGuire
The Green Seed Company
The Apple Barn
Rock Lane
Washington
West Sussex
Tel: 0181 789 7897
(organic seed supplies)

John Davidson
Wholistic Research Co.
The Old Forge
Mill Green
Hatfield
Hertfordshire AL9 5NZ
Tel: 01707 262686; fax: 01707 258828
(suppliers of juicers and health literature)

The FRESH Network
PO Box 71
Ely
Cambridgeshire CB7 4GU
Tel: 01353 662849
(lectures and seminars on vegetarianism based on 'living food' diets; quarterly membership magazine; juicing equipment and literature)

BIBLIOGRAPHY

Amazing Claims for Chlorophyll (Lowell), Nutrition Forum, 7/87.

Stephen Barrett, *Alternative Cancer Treatments*, Quackwatch website.

Stephen Barrett, *Antioxidants and Other Phytochemicals*, Quackwatch website, 1999.

Stephen Barrett, *The Dark Side of Linus Pauling's Legacy: Does Vitamin C Prevent Colds?*, Quackwatch website.

Stephen Barrett, *Dietary Supplements: Appropriate Use*, Quackwatch, website, 1999.

Stephen Barrett, *Gastronintestinal Quackery, Colonics, Laxatives, and More*, revised 20 July 1999, Quackwatch website.

Stephen Barrett, *Juicing*, Quackwatch website, 4 September 1999.

Stephen Barrett & Victor Herbert, *Questionable Cancer Therapies*, updated 20 September 1999.

Ruth Bircher-Benner, *Eating Your Way to Health*, Faber and Faber, 1961.

Stephen Blauer, *The Juicing Book*, Avery, NY, 1989.

Cherie Calbom & Maureen Keane, *Juicing for Life*, Avery Publishing Group, 1992.

Brian R. Clement & Theresa Foy Digeronimo, *Living Foods for Optimum Health*, Prima Health, 1998.

Vernon Coleman, *Eat Green, Lose Weight*, Angus & Robertson, 1990.

The Complete Raw Juice Therapy, Thorson, 1989.

The Composition of Food: Fruits and Nuts, Royal Society of Chemistry, issued by the Ministry of Agriculture and Fisheries, 1992.

The Composition of Food: Vegetable, Herbs and Spices, Royal Society of Chemistry, issued by the Ministry of Agriculture and Fisheries, 1992.

Alan Davidson, *The Oxford Companion of Food,* Oxford University Press, 1999.

John & Lucie Davidson, *A Harmony of Science and Nature,* Holistic Research Co., 1999.

Davidson, Passmore, Brock, Truswell, *Human Nutrition and Dietetics,* 7th edition, Churchill Livingstone, 1979.

Susan Dingott & Joanna Dwyer, *Vegetarianism: Healthful But Unnecessary,* article written in 1991, originally published in *Nutrition Forum*, Quackwatch website.

Fruit, a Connoisseur's Guide and Cookbook, Mitchell Beazley.

Pat Genry & Lynne Devereux, *Juice It Up,* 101 Productions, Santa Rosa, USA.

C. Hennekens, *Physicians Health Study II,* Harvard Medical School.

Dr Bernard Jensen, *Juicing Therapy,* Escondido, 1992.

Leslie Kenton with Russell Cronin, *Juice High,* Ebury Press, 1996.

Leslie Kenton, *Lean Revolution,* Ebury Press, 1994.

Leslie & Susannah Kenton, *Raw Energy*, Arrow, 1984.

Jethro Kloss, *Back to Eden,* Back to Eden Books, revised and expanded 1994.

Jay Kordich, *The Juiceman's Power of Juicing,* William Marrow and Co. Inc., NY, 1992.

William H. Lee, *The Book of Raw Fruit, Vegetable Juices and Drinks,* Keats, Conn., 1982.

William H. Lee, *Getting the Best Out of Your Juicer,* Keats, Conn., 1992.

Anne Lindsay, *The Low Risk Cancer Cookbook,* Grub Street, 1992.

Barry Lynch, *BBC Health Check,* BBC Books, 1989.

Leonard Mervyn, *Vitamins A, D and K,* Thorsons, 1984.

Morse, Rivers, Heughan, Barrie & Jenkins, *The Family Guide to Food and Health,* 1988.

National Council Against Health Fraud, *Wheatgrass Therapy:* C.1994, www.ncahf.org.

J.O. Rodale, *The Complete Book of Food and Nutrition*, Rodale Books Inc., Pennsylvania, 1972.

Jo Rogers, *The Encyclopedia of Food and Nutrition*, Merehurst, 1990.

Tom Sanders & Peter Bazalgette, *The Food Revolution*, Bantam Press, 1991.

Briony Thomas, *The Manual of Dietetic Practice*, edited by the British Dietetic Association, Blackwell Scientific Publications, 1988.

Unconventional Methods, a National Cancer Institute Fact Sheet, statement released October 1992, Quackwatch website.

Michael van Straten & Barbara Griggs, *Superfoods*, Dorling Kindersley, 1990.

N.W. Walker, *Become Younger*, Norwalk Press, Arizona, revised 1995.

N. W. Walker, *Colon Health: The Key to Vibrant Life*, Norwalk Press, Arizona,1979.

N.W. Walker, *Diet and Salad*, Norwalk Press, Arizona, 1986.

N.W. Walker, *Fresh Vegetable and Fruit Juices*, Norwalk Press, Arizona, 1978.

N.W. Walker, *The Natural Way to Vibrant Health*, Norwalk Press, Arizona, 1995.

Ruth Ward, *A Harvest of Apples*, Penguin, 1988.

What the Heck is Essiac, http://.members.oal.com/essiac/indexhtn.

Caroline Wheater, *Beta Carotene: How It Can Help Your Better Health*, Thorsons, 1991.

Caroline Wheater, *The Juicing Detox Diet*, Thorsons, 1993.

Caroline Wheater, *Juicing for Health*, Thorsons, 1993.

Ann Wigmore, *The Wheatgrass Book*, Avery Publishing Group Inc., Wayne, New Jersey, 1985.

Judith Wills, *Slim and Healthy Mediterranean*, Conran Octopus, 1992.

INDEX